Film-Screen Mammography

An Atlas of Instructional Cases

Film-Screen Mammography
An Atlas of Instructional Cases

Lawrence W Bassett, MD, FACR
Professor of Radiological Sciences
Director, The Iris Cantor Center for Breast Imaging

Reza Jahanshahi, MSIII
Post-Sophomore Fellow in Pathology

Richard H Gold, MD, FACR
Professor of Radiological Sciences
Chief of the Division of General Diagnosis

Yao S Fu, MD
Professor of Pathology

UCLA School of Medicine and the Jonsson Comprehensive Cancer Center at UCLA, Los Angeles, California

RAVEN PRESS   **MARTIN DUNITZ**

First published in the USA in 1991
by Raven Press, New York, NY

First published in the United Kingdom in 1991
by Martin Dunitz, 7–9 Pratt Street, London NW1 0AE

Library of Congress Cataloging-in-Publication Data

90-63208

ISBN 0-88167-756-6

Typeset by Scribe Design, Gillingham, Kent
Origination by Adroit Photolitho Ltd, Birmingham
Printed and bound in England by the University Press, Cambridge

Contents

Acknowledgment

The authors thank Mary Frazier, their tireless Administrative Assistant.

Preface

The field of breast imaging is undergoing rapid improvements in technology and a tremendous increase in utilization. Mammography is now recognized as the most effective technique for the detection of early breast cancer, and film-screen mammography has become the most widely used method. The increasing use of film-screen mammography has resulted in a demand by mammographers for additional teaching tools, particularly for diagnostic decision making.

Following an introductory chapter, this Atlas provides an opportunity for its readers to test their skills in interpreting the mammograms of a wide variety of pathologically proven cases. The cases were selected on the basis of their diversity of mammographic manifestations, with their emphasis on the often subtle features of carcinoma.

Each case begins with a short history, followed by mammograms for self-testing. In order to make them more realistic, the test mammograms have been reproduced to full size and are free of arrows or other indicators of the location of abnormalities. Although some of the mammograms were photographed so that their representations were as close to the originals as possible, others were photographed so as to enhance the visibility of specific findings, and in these images the skin line is frequently not visible. Readers may find a magnifying lens useful when looking at these mammograms, just as they would at the view box.

For each case, the test mammograms are bounded by coordinate grids made up of letters on one axis and numbers on the other, to locate abnormalities that are described in the next section, 'Findings'. The 'Discussion' section which follows includes additional mammograms, results of the diagnostic workup, clinical follow-up, surgical and pathologic findings, and important relevant issues. Pathologic correlation has been provided for the majority of cases.

The book covers, in summary form, the important topics found in the mammography literature today; a large number of references are provided for additional reading.

LWB
RJ
RHG
YSF

Introduction to Mammography and Breast Cancer Screening

Breast cancer continues to be the most common cancer of American women, and its incidence is increasing. In the US in 1990 an estimated 150 000 new cases will be diagnosed, and 44 000 women will die of the disease.[137] The mortality rate for breast cancer in the US has remained unchanged for the past 50 years and is similar to that of any Western industrialized nation.[137] The greatest risk is for women over age 40, and the incidence progressively increases until age 70. The best hope for improved survival is early detection of clinically occult cancer by screening.

The most successful method of breast cancer screening is mammography. Its success encompasses both earlier detection and decreased mortality.[11] It is estimated that, on average, a mammogram can detect a breast cancer 2 years before it is palpable. The first randomized controlled study of screening mammography was undertaken by the Health Insurance Plan (HIP) of Greater New York from 1963–6.[126] Women were offered annual screening by physical examination and mammography for 4 successive years. After 7 years, there was a 30 percent reduction in breast cancer mortality in the women offered screening compared to those in the control group. After 18 years, the mortality was still reduced by 23 percent. If mammography had been omitted from the annual screening, the benefit probably would have fallen by one-third.

The Breast Cancer Detection Demonstration Project (BCDDP) was sponsored by the American Cancer Society (ACS) and the National Cancer Institute (NCI).[11] From 1973–8, 280 000 women were scheduled to undergo 5 consecutive annual screenings using physical examination and mammography. As this was a demonstration project, and not a controlled study, definitive conclusions about the value of screening could not be derived from the data. However, the results implied that mammography had undergone a vast improvement since the HIP study. Mammography detected 91 percent of the cancers in the BCDDP. Of these, 42 percent were detected only with

mammography, compared with 33 percent in the HIP study. On the other hand, 9 percent of cancers were detected only by physical examination, compared with 44 percent in the HIP study. None of the cancers detected by screening in the HIP study was less than 1 cm, whereas one-third of all BCDDP cancers were noninfiltrating, or infiltrating but less than 1 cm in size, and most of these were detected by mammography alone. Less than 20 percent of all the cancers detected in the BCDDP had spread to the axillary lymph nodes.[11] This is one-half the rate of nodal involvement associated with newly diagnosed breast cancers in the general population.

Several studies from Europe have confirmed the value of mammographic screening. The first was a Dutch case-control study where all women over 35 in Nijmegen were invited to participate in single-view mammography every 2 years from 1975–81.[150] As a result of screening, mortality from breast cancer was reduced by 52 percent. A second Dutch case-control study, at Utrecht, involved women aged 50–64, who were screened initially, then at 12, 18, and 24 months.[27] In this study, mortality from breast cancer was decreased by 70 percent. A population-based randomized control study in Sweden began in 1977 with single-view screening mammograms at 24- to 33-month intervals. After 7 years, there was a 31 percent decrease in mortality as well as 25 percent fewer stage II and greater cancers in the women who were screened.[144]

Performing the examination

Film-screen mammography has three primary views: mediolateral oblique, lateral and cephalocaudal (Figure I.1a,b,c). Clinical investigations have identified the mediolateral oblique projection as the most effective single view.[8,13,92] The superiority of this view is due to the fact that it

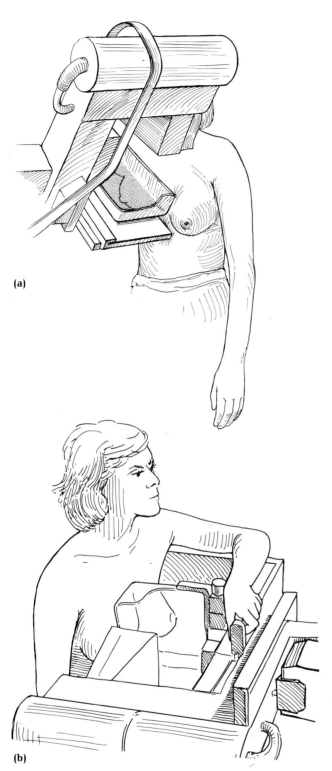

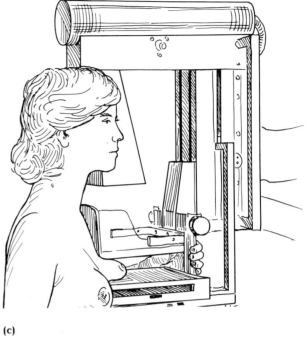

Figure I.1

Positioning for film-screen mammography. (a)
Mediolateral oblique view. Breast is distracted from the
pectoralis major muscle and compressed at an angle
parallel to the plane of the muscle. (b) Lateral view. This
view can be performed either mediolateral or
lateromedial. The mediolateral view is shown here. The
patient is rotated slightly inward, and the arm is
supported by the C-arm of the dedicated unit.
(c) Cephalocaudal view.

most completely depicts the deeper structures of
the upper–outer quadrant and axillary tail. It is
obtained by directing the X-ray beam perpendicu-
lar to the pectoralis major muscle in a supero-
medial to inferolateral direction. The lateral view
is obtained with the X-ray beam directed from
medial to lateral, or lateral to medial, with compression applied in the true lateral plane. The
lateral view is used in conjunction with the
cephalocaudal view to determine in three dimen-
sions the exact location of a lesion. In the cephalocaudal view, the X-ray beam is directed 90
degrees from the lateral, with compression
applied parallel to the floor.

Some investigators have suggested the use of
single-view screening examinations to reduce
radiation exposure, cost and examination time.[93]
Others have found that the rate of cancer detection is too low with single-view examinations. A
major limitation of single-view screening is that a
cancer may be obscured by overlying parenchymal tissue in one projection, yet visible in

another.[8,106] Furthermore, single-view screening may actually be less cost-effective than two-view screening since greater numbers of patients need to be called back for additional views after single-view examinations.[12,136]

In a recent study, oblique, lateral and cephalo-caudal views were done on 9662 patients.[12] Of 172 cancers found in these patients, 125 (72.7 percent) were seen on all three views, 11 (6.4 percent) on the oblique view only, 4 (2.3 percent) on the lateral only and 3 (1.7 percent) on the cephalocaudal view only. Ten cancers (5.8 percent) were not depicted on any view. Two-view mediolateral oblique-cephalocaudal mammograms showed 158 (91.9 percent) of 172 cancers, and mediolateral-cephalocaudal combinations showed 151 (87.8 percent).

Adequate breast compression is essential for high-quality mammograms. Compression holds the breast still, preventing motion, separates tissues to disclose small lesions, improves image quality and reduces radiation dose by decreasing breast thickness.[41] Recent studies show that the compression required for mammography is acceptable to patients when they know its importance, and will not cause them to refuse mammography.[140]

Special views are used to better define a lesion or verify its presence. Examples are exaggerated cephalocaudal views *(Figure I.2a)* and spot (coned) compression *(Figure I.2c)* applied over a local area of interest.[18]

The normal breast

Embryology

In the sixth week of fetal development, epidermal thickenings appear bilaterally along the mammary lines, extending from the axillae to the groin.[10] In humans the epidermal thickenings disappear shortly after their formation and only a small portion in the thoracic region persists. Cords of cells grow downwards from the base of the epidermis producing small, solid outbuddings which later form lumina giving rise to rudimentary branching ducts. After birth, progressive growth and branching of these ducts continue at a very slow pace until puberty. At this stage development of the breast ceases in the male. In the female, with the onset of menstruation, the growth rate increases with branching of the ducts and

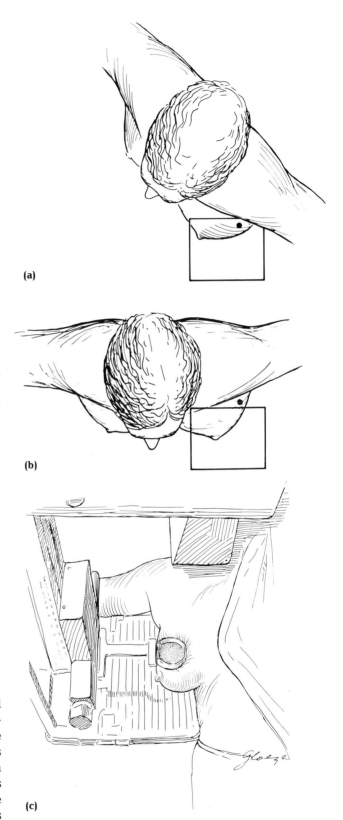

(a)

(b)

(c)

Figure I.2

Special views. (**a**) Exaggerated cephalocaudal view. A lesion in the outer quadrant, near the axilla, is not imaged in the routine cephalocaudal view (**b**). The patient is rotated, and the exaggerated outer cephalocaudal includes the lesion. (**c**) Spot compression.

proliferation of the interductal stroma. At the same time the terminal ducts give rise to small, blind, grape-like outpouchings, the rudimentary gland buds.

Anatomy and histology

The base of the breast extends from the second to sixth rib in the midclavicular line over the pectoralis major muscle. The glandular tissue always spreads further than the gross outline of the breast. Commonly, a long tongue-like process of breast tissue, the axillary appendage, or tail of Spence, extends from the main mass up the anterior axillary line towards and even into the axilla.[3] This is of considerable importance, since it may give rise to benign or malignant abnormalities that may be mistaken for pathology of the axillary lymph nodes.

Histologically, the female breast consists of 15–20 lobes of glandular tissue whose associated ducts, the lactiferous ducts, extend to approximately 8 orifices at the nipple *(Figure I.3)*.[109] Each

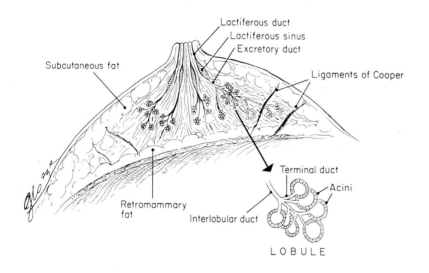

Figure I.3

Schematic diagram of mature breast in axial section.

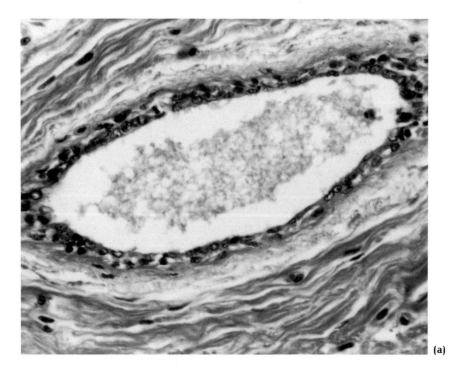

(a)

Figure I.4

Histology of mature breast.
(a) The normal duct is made up of two layers of cells, an inner epithelial layer and outer myoepithelial layer.
(b) Interlobular duct (arrow), terminal ducts (arrowhead) and acini making up the lobule.
(c) Acini.

lactiferous duct enlarges immediately behind the aerola to form a lactiferous sinus, in which milk and other secretions can accumulate. Beyond the lactiferous sinuses the ducts branch and rebranch, ending in terminal ducts or ductules *(Figure I.4a,b)*. Each of the terminal ducts gives rise to a small saccular gland or acinus which is the milk-producing unit of the breast *(Figure I.4c)*. The functional glandular unit of the mammary gland, the lobule, is composed of an interlobular duct, terminal ducts (ductules) and associated acini. During lactation, the terminal ducts and acini

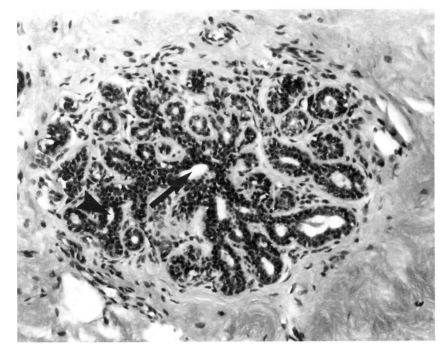

(b)

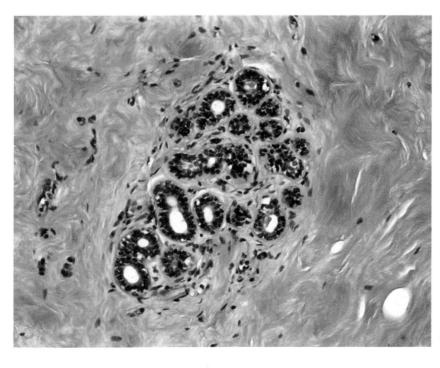

(c)

undergo hyperplasia and secretory activity. There is some disagreement over the use of the term 'acinus'. Some apply the term to signify the terminal units during the resting stage, while others limit it to the secretory units of lactating breast tissue. During the resting phase, acini may become inconspicuous and the lobules are then comprised largely of terminal ducts.[151] When the acini become dilated, they are indistinguishable from ductules.

Under low-power histologic examination, two basic units are distinguished: lobules and ducts. Much of the terminology for breast pathology is based on this distinction. The acini, ductules and ducts are lined by inner secretory cells and outer myoepithelial cells *(Figure I.4a)*. The myofilaments in the latter cells provide contractility to squeeze the secretory products towards the nipple. The glandular tissue is embedded in a mass of fibrous and adipose tissue.

The breast derives its structural support from dense fibrous tissue septae, the ligaments of Cooper, bands of which extend from the deep fascia over the pectoralis major muscle to the dermis *(Figure 1.3)*. Sometimes carcinoma of the breast calls attention to itself by retracting the ligaments so as to produce dimpling of the skin.

Knowledge of the lymphatic drainage of the breast is important because of its frequent involvement with carcinoma. The axillary lymph nodes normally receive more than 75 percent of the total drainage. Other routes of lymphatic drainage include the supraclavicular, interpectoral and internal mammary lymph nodes.

Breast pathology

This section reviews the pathologic terminology used in this Atlas. A more detailed discussion of pathology is presented with the individual cases.

Fibroadenoma, a benign localized proliferation of both ductal and stromal components, is the commonest neoplasm detected during the second and third decades of life. Degenerative changes, common in older lesions, include fibrosis, hyalinization, calcification of the stroma, and calcification within the ducts of the tumor. Infarction of fibroadenoma occasionally occurs post partum. The epithelial cells of a fibroadenoma may undergo proliferation, atrophy or fibrocystic change. Rarely, intraductal and lobular carcinoma in situ may occur in fibroadenoma, with or without additional lesions elsewhere. The malignant counterpart of fibroadenoma is cystosarcoma phyllodes, in which the stroma undergoes sarcoma-

tous transformation. Benign phyllodes tumors may also occur.

Intraductal papilloma arises from large interlobular and excretory ducts, and predominates in the subareolar region. Epithelial cells proliferate in a complex finger-like pattern supported by a fibrovascular core. With time, the process extends into the smaller branching ducts, resulting in multiple nodules on low-power microscopy. Secretory products admixed with blood from an infarcted papilloma lead to a bloody nipple discharge. Degenerative changes of the supporting stalk can lead to fibrosis, hyalinization, calcification and distorted ducts simulating invasive carcinoma.

In reproductive and perimenopausal women, the most common breast changes are related to imbalanced hormonal stimulation, and are characterized by adenosis, epithelial proliferation and fibrocystic changes, which often coexist. Fibrocystic changes affect primarily the ductal segments. The ducts become dilated and cystic, and contain serous or turbid fluid. The epithelial lining of the cysts may be absent, flattened or hyperplastic. Apocrine metaplasia and papillary proliferation are common. Inflammatory responses surrounding the cysts are usually chronic and mild.

Adenosis refers to epithelial proliferation of the lobules. Lactational change is a form of adenosis. In nonlactating women, the early phase of adenosis is characterized by an enlargement of the lobules caused by a marked increase of acini and ductules. Subsequently, proliferation of myoepithelial cells and sclerosis of the stroma cause the lobular architecture to become irregular and distorted. This phase is referred to as 'sclerosing adenosis'. The end result is atrophy. Calcifications within foci of adenosis usually take the form of small laminated bodies in the acini and less commonly in the stroma. Multiple lobules of adenosis can form a discrete gross tumor, designated by Haagensen as an adenosis tumor.[54]

Epithelial hyperplasia, as classified by Page, is divided into lobular (when proliferation occurs within the lobules), and ductal (when it is outside of the lobules).[109] This distinction is usually made by low-power microscopic observation. The 'usual' ductal hyperplasia is graded as mild, moderate or florid. The morphologic hallmark of epithelial hyperplasia is increased cellularity and altered architecture, most commonly with papillary formation, a sieve-like cribriform pattern and cellular filling of the lumens. These changes are also referred to as 'epitheliosis' and 'papillomatosis'.

In the presence of architectural and nuclear atypia, the hyperplasia is designated as atypical ductal hyperplasia or atypical lobular hyperplasia. These atypical hyperplasias have some but not all the morphologic features of an in-situ carcinoma. The atypical lesions contain proliferating cells with enlarged, irregular, hyperchromatic nuclei, and nucleoli. They are intermingled with the normal secretory or myoepithelial cells, thus giving the appearance of heterogeneity. In a ductal or lobular carcinoma in situ, the involved focus is occupied by a homogeneous population of neoplastic cells.

The system of nomenclature proposed by Page[108,109] has the advantage of correlating pathologic changes with the risk of developing invasive breast cancer. In comparison to the general population, there is no significant increase of risk for women with nonproliferative changes, such as regular, sclerosing or florid adenosis, apocrine change, ductal ectasia or mild epithelial hyperplasia of the usual type. A slight increase of relative risk, in the range of 1.5–2 times, is noted for women with moderate or florid hyperplasia without atypia. The relative risk is increased to 4–5 times among women with atypical ductal or atypical lobular hyperplasia, and 8–10 times for ductal or lobular carcinoma in situ.[108]

By the above criteria, 70 percent of biopsies of fibrocystic changes are nonproliferative lesions, 26 percent are proliferative without atypia, and 4 percent are proliferative with atypia.[36] Within the epithelial proliferative lesions, stromal fibrosis, elastosis and hyalinization produce stellate-shaped, indurated lesions. The entrapped, distorted ducts, especially adjacent to adenosis and papillary lesions, can be confused with invasive carcinoma histologically. These lesions are known by different terms, including sclerosing papillary proliferation,[44] indurative mastopathy[115] and radial scar.[89] They can result in gross architectural distortions that may mimic malignancy on mammograms.

Breast carcinomas are generally believed to progress from carcinoma in situ to early invasive carcinoma and then to frankly invasive carcinoma. This stepwise progression is apparent among women undergoing mammographic screening. In one study of 62 nonpalpable breast cancers detected by mammography, there were 20 (32 percent) ductal carcinomas in situ, 5 (8 percent) lobular carcinomas in situ, 7 (11 percent) minimal invasive ductal carcinomas and 30 (48 percent) invasive ductal carcinomas.[125] Thus, mammographic screening detected almost 50 percent of breast cancers at an early, potentially curable, in-situ or early invasive stage. However, relatively few American women with breast cancers are detected at the early stages possible with mammographic screening. In a survey of 24 000 new breast cancers in 1978, only 0.84 percent were

ductal carcinomas in situ.[120] Of the 2072 stage I and II breast cancer specimens studied by the National Surgical Adjuvant Breast Project (NSABP), only 78 (3.8 percent) were ductal carcinoma in situ.[47]

Breast carcinomas are classified histologically into ductal and lobular types. Each type is further divided into in-situ and invasive categories on the basis of stromal invasion. In intraductal or in-situ ductal carcinoma, the malignant cells proliferate within the existing ductal system without destruction of the surrounding basement membrane. They form complex papillary projections, cribriform patterns or solid nests. The latter are typically seen in the comedo variant characterized by central necrosis of the intraductal tumor leading to calcification within the involved ducts. Malignant cells spread along the existing ducts causing multifocal disease, Paget's disease of the nipple, and 'cancerization' of the lobules.

The cells of invasive ductal carcinoma break through the duct wall and invade the stroma, adjacent breast tissue and, eventually, the lymphatic channels. Intraductal carcinoma may persist in the earliest stage as the predominant component, but with time the invasive component comes to predominate, leaving few or no in-situ foci.

The majority of invasive ductal carcinomas are of the 'not otherwise specified' type, with heterogeneous microscopic patterns. Mucinous (colloid), papillary, tubular and medullary carcinomas are special variants of ductal carcinoma that have a distinct morphology and more favorable prognosis than the not-otherwise-specified variant.[45,48] Inflammatory carcinoma is also recognized as a distinct entity because of its characteristic clinical presentation, dermal lymphatic invasion and dismal outcome.

Lobular carcinoma in situ is characterized by filling of the lobules with relatively small, uniform cells. Invasive lobular carcinoma has a tendency to spread diffusely between collagen fibers. This results in tumor cells arranged in a single layer, the so-called Indian-file pattern. The individual cells have small, round nuclei and scanty cytoplasm.

Rare breast carcinomas include secretory carcinoma, adenoid cystic carcinoma, squamous cell carcinoma, and metaplastic carcinoma. Nonepithelial tumors rarely occur in the breast. Some of these are granular cell tumor, stromal cell sarcoma, lymphoma, hemangioma and angiosarcoma. Finally, extramammary malignancies may metastasize to the breast.

Some non-neoplastic conditions can present clinically with a breast mass and simulate neoplastic lesions clinically and mammographically. Some of these are common lesions, such as mammary duct ectasia, fibrous mastopathy and fat necrosis, and will be discussed in this Atlas.

The normal mammogram

The breasts of adolescent women are usually radiopaque because they are composed primarily of dense fibroglandular tissue. This radiopacity limits the accuracy of mammographic examinations.[42] With increasing age and after childbearing, the dense glandular tissue is replaced by radiolucent fat in which abnormalities are more readily detected (Figure I.5a,b). Normally, the breast is relatively symmetrical bilaterally. Surgery, fibrocystic changes and desmoplastic response to carcinoma can result in asymmetry. In order to detect subtle asymmetry, the mammograms should be viewed such that the right and left breasts can be compared.

Mammographic features of malignant and benign diseases

The mammographic features of malignancy can be divided into primary, secondary and indirect signs. The primary signs of malignancy include a mass, often of relatively high radiographic density, and/or microcalcifications. Secondary signs, such as skin thickening and retraction, are usually clinically obvious. Subtle indirect signs may be the only evidence of nonpalpable cancer and include architectural distortion, parenchymal asymmetry, a unilateral focus of one or more prominent ducts, and a developing neodensity.[7,96,104,127]

Prebiopsy needle localization

Mammographically guided prebiopsy needle localization is indicated for any occult lesion, defined as any suspicious lesion seen in mammograms but not identified on clinical examination. The purpose of prebiopsy needle localization is to ensure removal of an occult lesion with the smallest possible breast deformity.

Variations of needle localization include: (1) the direct needle approach where the tip of a hypodermic needle is inserted as close as possible to the abnormality and left in place when the patient goes to surgery,[146] (2) a 'spot' method which involves injecting methylene blue dye ($0.1 \, cm^3$) through the properly positioned needle prior to removing the needle,[37] and (3) the most reliable method, a needle-wire assembly consisting of a needle containing a malleable wire with a barbed or rounded hook at the end.[67,76]

After needle localization, specimen radiography should be performed on every surgical specimen—even those without calcification—to confirm the presence of the lesion and to enhance histologic sampling of the suspicious areas.

Fine-needle aspiration biopsy

Fine-needle aspiration biopsy is useful to evaluate some palpable and nonpalpable mammographically localized lesions that might be carcinomas or fibroadenomas. Should the cystological findings be inconclusive or negative, surgical biopsy is required.

False-negative mammograms

Approximately 10–15 percent of carcinomas cannot be detected on mammograms. Treatment of a palpable carcinoma may be adversely affected when a biopsy is delayed because of a negative mammogram. In one study, 36 women with breast masses and negative mammograms were eventually shown to have biopsy-proven malignancy.[95] Of the 17 women who had biopsies performed within 2 months of their negative mammograms, 17.6 percent had extension to the axillary nodes. Of the 19 who had biopsies delayed from 3–24 months (mean 12 months), 59.7 percent had axillary node involvement. Thus mammography cannot be considered a substitute for biopsy in the presence of suspicious clinical findings.

Breast sonography

The breast was one of the first organs examined by ultrasound.[152] Breast sonography has at various times been promoted for cancer screening.[26,73] However, sensitivity and specificity of breast sonography for the detection of breast

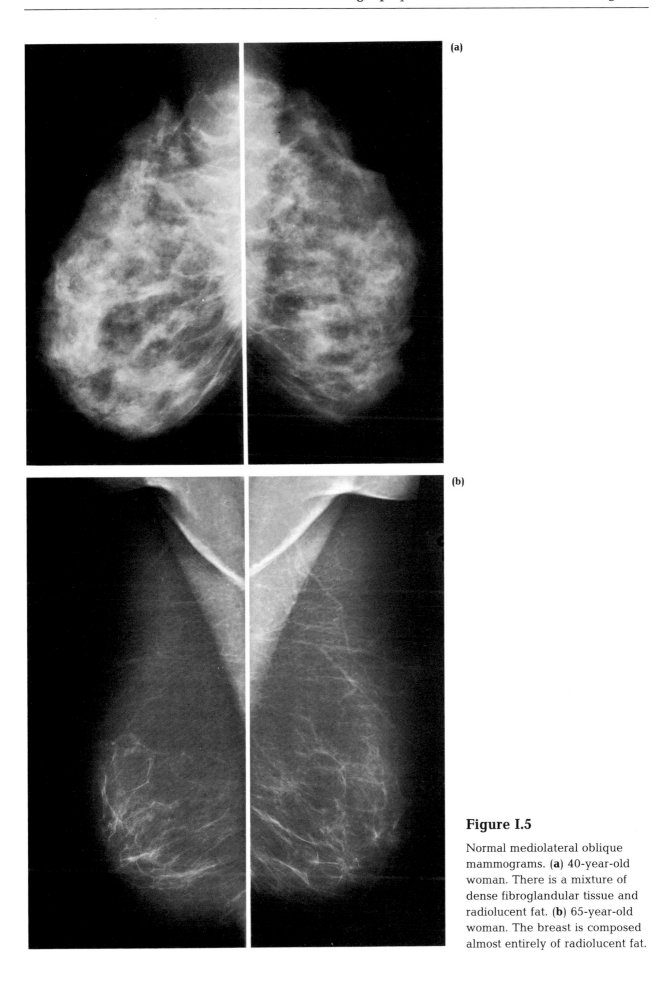

(a)

(b)

Figure I.5

Normal mediolateral oblique mammograms. (**a**) 40-year-old woman. There is a mixture of dense fibroglandular tissue and radiolucent fat. (**b**) 65-year-old woman. The breast is composed almost entirely of radiolucent fat.

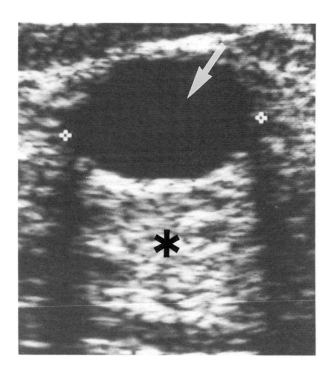

Figure I.6

Cyst. Sonographic features include smooth anterior and posterior boundaries, anechoic interior (arrow) and enhanced through transmission of sound (asterisk). Cursors are used to make direct measurement of cyst size.

cancer is far lower than state-of-the-art mammography.[16,78,131] The limitations of ultrasound include: (1) poor results with fatty breasts; (2) inability to depict microcalcifications; (3) inconsistent detection of solid lesions under 1 cm in diameter; and (4) unreliable criteria for differentiation between benign and malignant solid masses.

Today, breast sonography is most often used to differentiate cystic from solid masses found by palpation or on mammograms, with reported accuracy rates of 96–100 percent.[61,132] Sonography is the only reliable method to make cyst/solid differentiation of a small, nonpalpable, mammographically detected mass for which aspiration is likely to be unsuccessful.

Sonography can detect cysts as small as 2 mm. Cysts are the most frequent breast masses in women between the ages of 35 and 50. They can be solitary or multiple. Sonographic features include well-circumscribed anterior and posterior boundaries, round or oval shape, anechoic interior, and enhanced echoes distal to the cyst[61] *(Figure I.6)*. Of these features, an anechoic interior is the most diagnostic.

Cases

Case 1

A 71-year-old woman had a firm mass in the left breast.

Film: Cephalocaudal view of the left breast *(Figure 1.1)*.

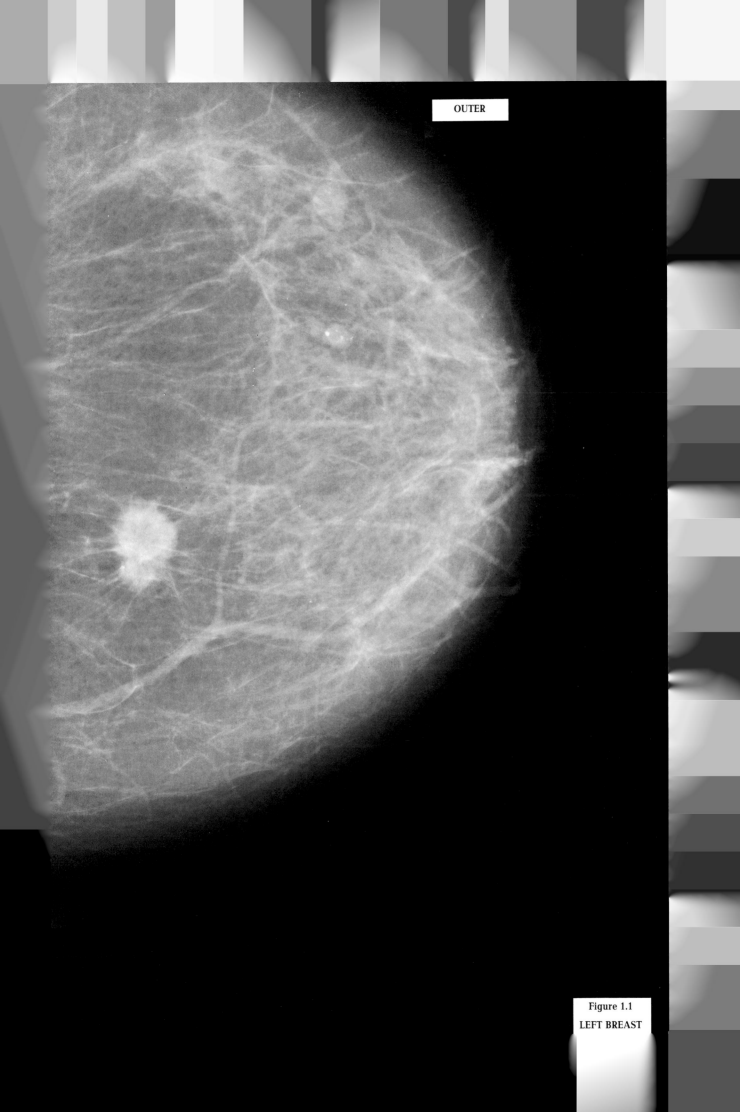

OUTER

Figure 1.1
LEFT BREAST

Findings

Seen in the breast are a 2.5 by 1.5 cm dense, spiculated mass (J7) and two small, lobulated, well-circumscribed, low-density masses (M2,M4), one of which has coarse calcification.

Discussion

The well-circumscribed masses were felt to represent benign degenerating fibroadenomas. The larger palpable mass is dense and has an irregular, spiculated margin typical of carcinoma. A biopsy of the palpable mass revealed moderately differentiated infiltrating ductal carcinoma *(Figures 1.2, 1.3)*.

Mammographically, the margins of a tumor mass are perhaps the most important feature for its differential diagnosis.[52] Infiltrating carcinomas are characterized by a distinct central tumor mass and irregular, sometimes spiculated, margins. The spicules of infiltrating carcinoma tend to extend in all directions from the central tumor mass, whereas the spicules occasionally associated with benign conditions, such as fibrocystic changes, tend to be bunched together in parallel rays like the straw in a broom.[143]

Infiltrating carcinomas are accompanied frequently by a desmoplastic reaction, a proliferation of fibrous tissue in and around the tumor, that causes them to become hard and fixed to the surrounding tissues. The nature and purpose of this host response is not understood, although it is postulated that specific factors released by the tumor are responsible for it.[58] Because on clinical examination these desmoplastic tumors seem to be larger than they appear to be in the mammogram, the mammogram provides a more accurate assessment of their size.[121] The desmoplastic reaction can thicken and shorten adjacent Cooper's ligaments, resulting in skin retraction, especially when the tumor is located superficially. Similarly, carcinomas in the subareolar area can produce thickening and shortening of the ducts, resulting in nipple retraction.

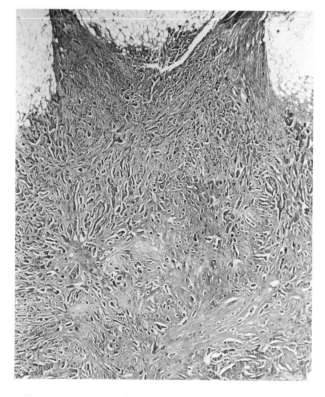

Figure 1.2

Low-power histologic section. In addition to its malignant epithelial cells, the tumor is composed of a large amount of fibrous tissue. There is an irregular boundary between the carcinoma and the surrounding mammary fat.

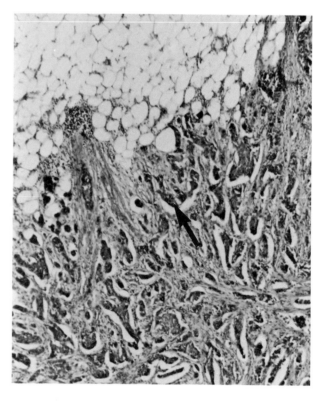

Figure 1.3

High-power histologic section. There is infiltration of mammary fat by small nests of tumor cells (arrow) and fibrous tendrils producing the irregular boundary observed in the mammogram. **Diagnosis**: Infiltrating ductal carcinoma.

Case 2

This 47-year-old woman felt a small movable lump in the right breast.

Films: Right *(Figure 2.1)* and left *(Figure 2.2)* mediolateral oblique mammograms.

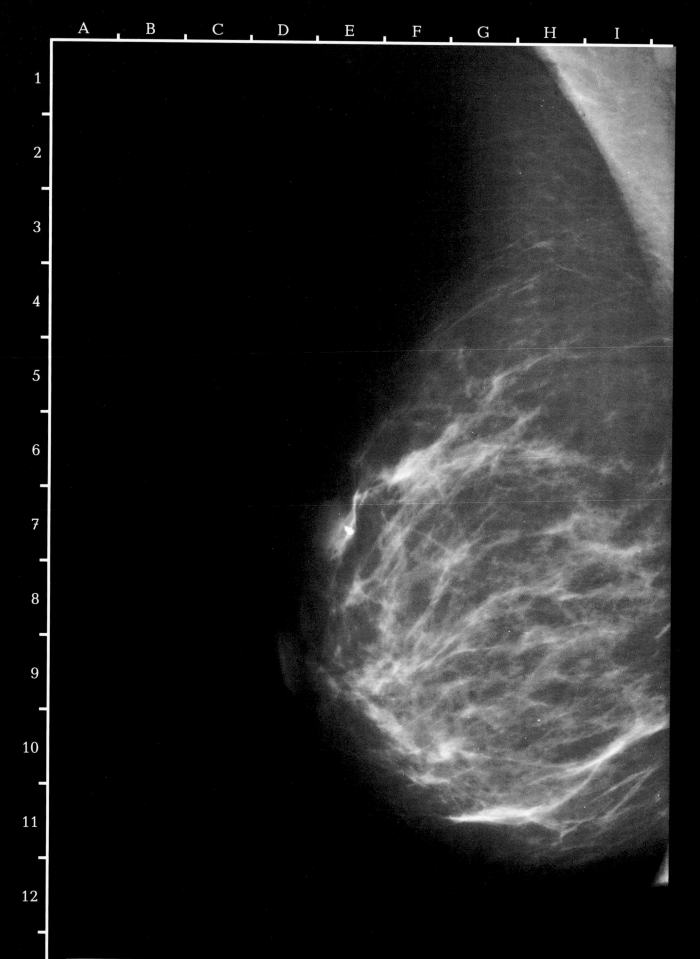

Figure 2.1
RIGHT BREAST

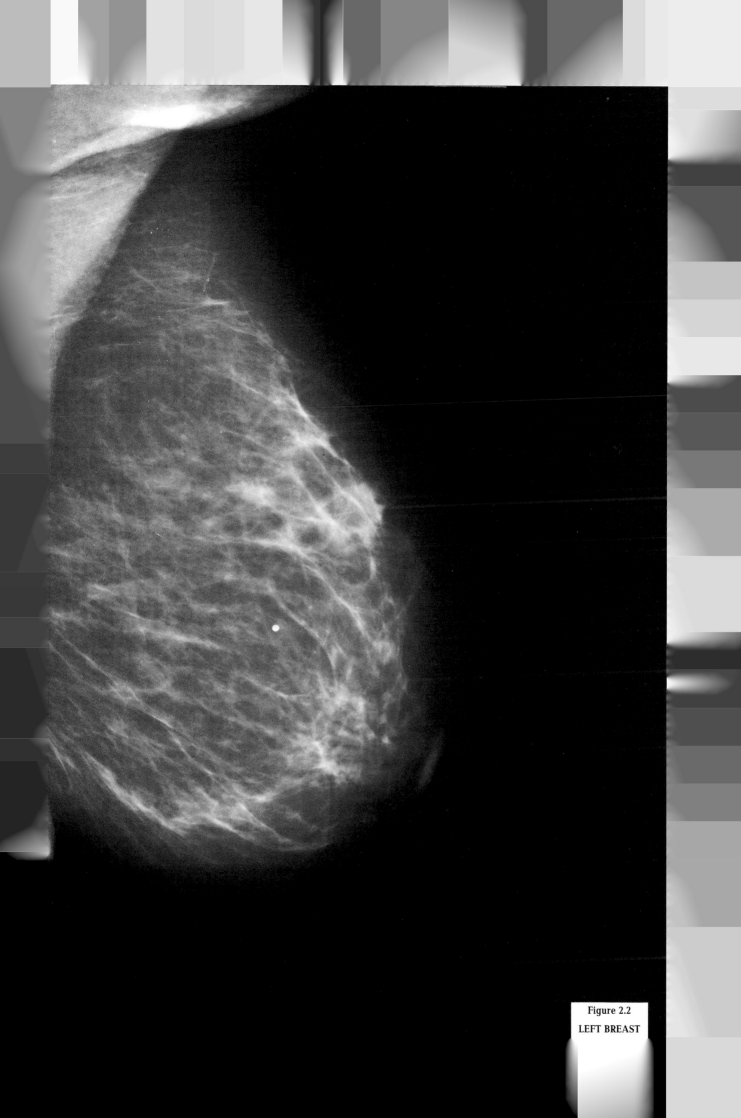

Figure 2.2
LEFT BREAST

Findings

There is a relatively well circumscribed 1.5 cm low-density mass containing a coarse calcification (E7) in the upper hemisphere of the right breast. There is a similar low-density mass without calcifications in the left breast (N6). A solitary coarse calcification with a relatively radiolucent center is present in the center of the left breast (L8).

Discussion

Cephalocaudal views *(Figures 2.3 and 2.4)* confirmed the low density and smooth margins of the masses and aided in their localization. The mammographic impression was benign masses, probably fibroadenomas. A biopsy performed on the palpable mass in the right breast showed a fibroadenoma *(Figures 2.5 and 2.6)*.

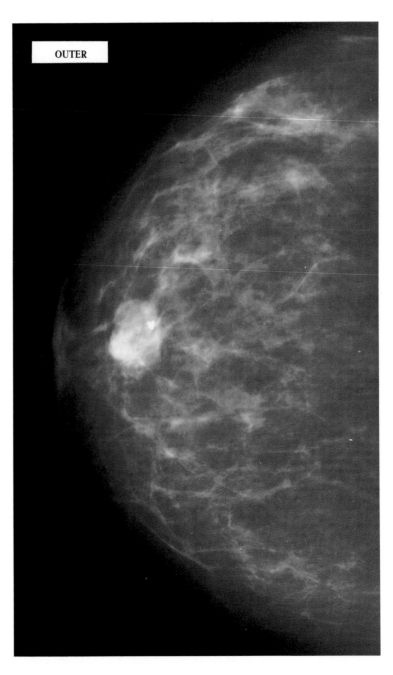

OUTER

Figure 2.3

Cephalocaudal mammogram of right breast. The well-circumscribed, calcified mass is posterior to the nipple.

Fibroadenomas are the most common breast masses seen in women under age 35. They are believed to arise from stromal and epithelial proliferation associated with estrogenic stimulation. Mammographically, they are typically well circumscribed, oval or lobulated. In postmenopausal women, fibroadenomas undergo atrophy and frequently calcify, as in this case. The calcifications of fibroadenomas are typically coarse and sharply marginated. Although there are rare reports of lobular carcinoma in situ arising in fibroadenomas, the latter are almost always benign.[98] The benign-appearing mass in the contralateral breast has been followed with annual mammograms for several years and has remained stable.

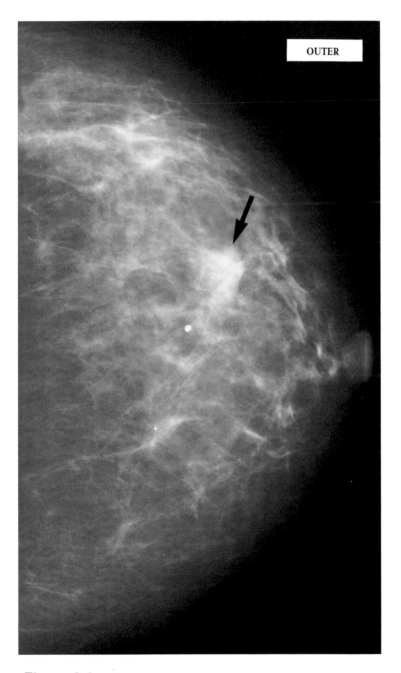

Figure 2.4

Cephalocaudal mammogram of left breast. The low-density mass (arrow) is slightly lateral to the nipple.

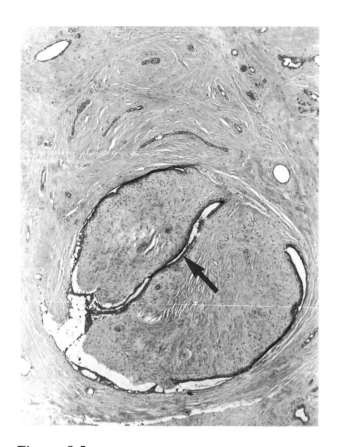

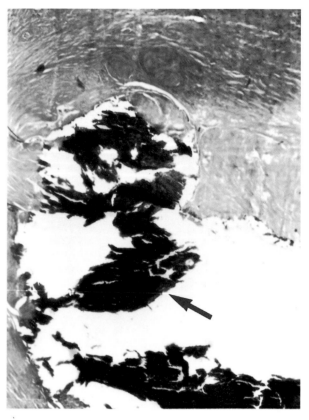

Figure 2.5

Low-power histologic section shows typical features of fibroadenoma: fibrous proliferation of stroma with compression of ducts (arrow).

Figure 2.6

Calcification (arrow) fills a dilated, atrophied ductal structure.

Case 3

This 67-year-old woman was referred for a screening mammogram.

Films: Right *(Figure 3.1)* and left *(Figure 3.2)* cephalocaudal mammograms.

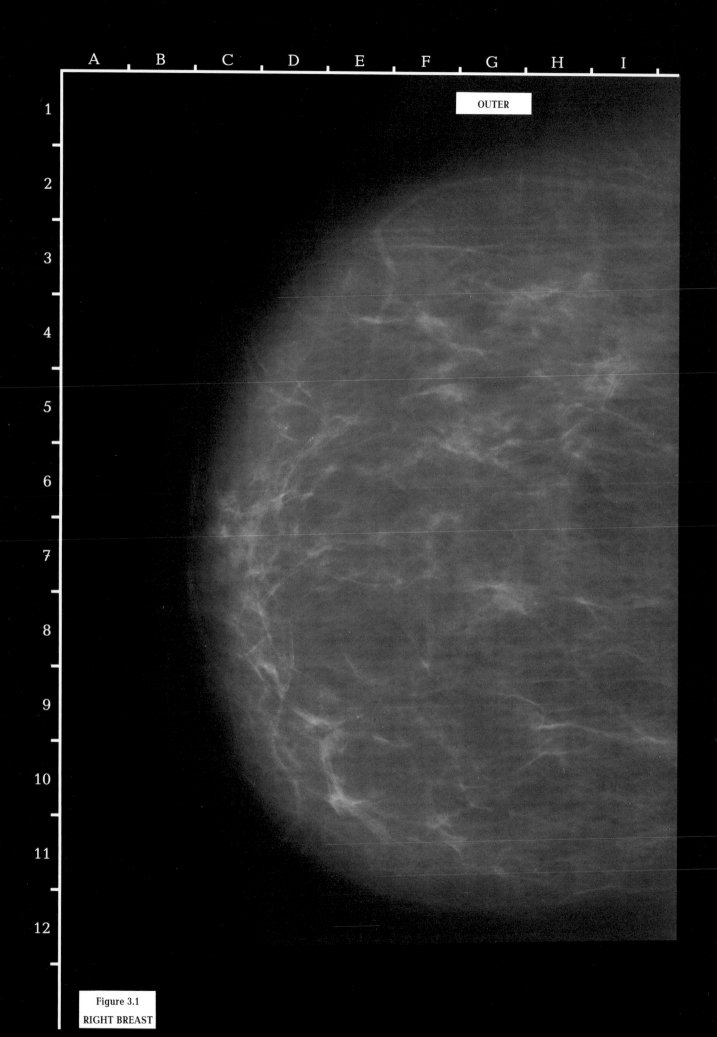

OUTER

Figure 3.1
RIGHT BREAST

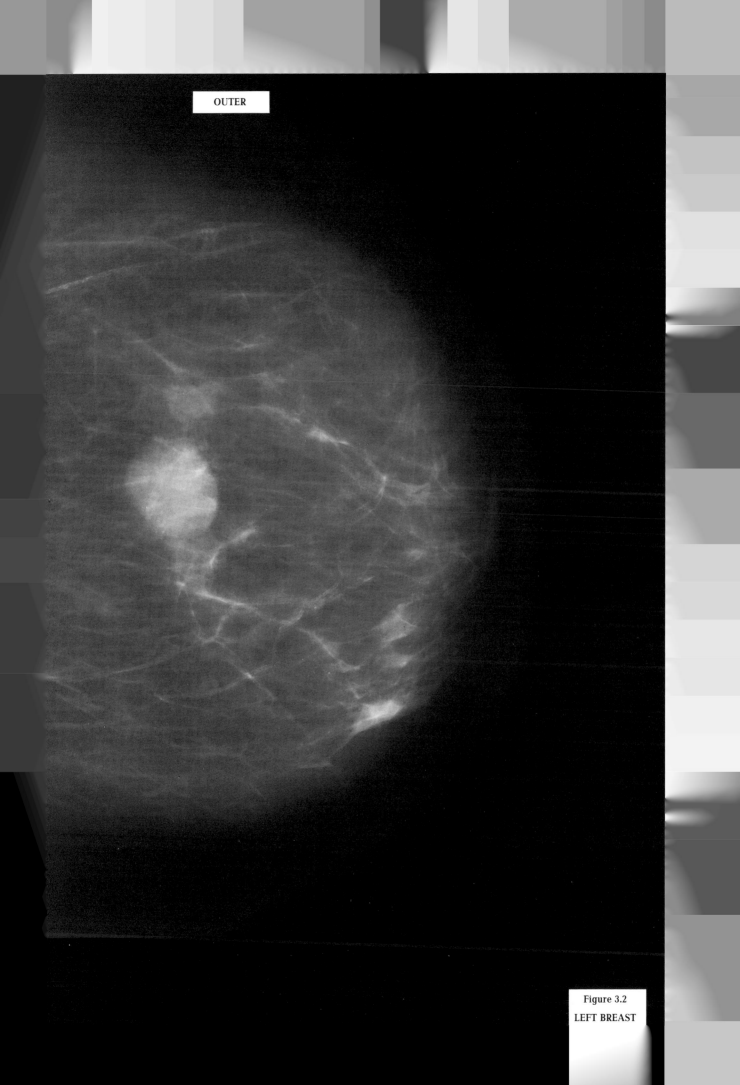

OUTER

OUTER

Figure 3.2
LEFT BREAST

Findings

There is a dominant mass (K6) in the left breast. There are two areas of arterial calcification in the left breast (J4 and M8).

Discussion

Because the mass has smooth margins, the possibility of a cyst was considered. Sonography revealed an anechoic mass with enhanced through transmission, typical of a cyst *(Figure 3.3)*.[61] However, in one section of the sonogram there appeared to be a nodule in the cyst wall *(Figure 3.4)*, raising the possibility of intracystic carcinoma. Therefore, a pneumocystogram was performed by aspiration of the cyst fluid and injection of air into the evacuated cyst. The pneumocystogram revealed a bilobed cyst, and the smooth inner walls indicated that no tumor was present *(Figures 3.5 and 3.6)*.[145] The cyst fluid was clear and showed no malignant cells by cytologic examination. The nodule in the sonogram was determined to represent part of the septum between the two compartments of the cyst.

Intracystic carcinoma is rare.[29] Of 434 pneumocystograms reported by Tabár, 26 (6 percent) revealed either benign or malignant intracystic tumors.[145] He reported that neither visual nor cytologic examination of the fluid alone was sufficient to detect or rule out intracystic carcinoma. Without evidence of intracystic tumor on pneumocystography, cyst removal is unnecessary. According to Tabár, pneumocystography is therapeutic in that it aids in preventing the recurrence of the cyst.

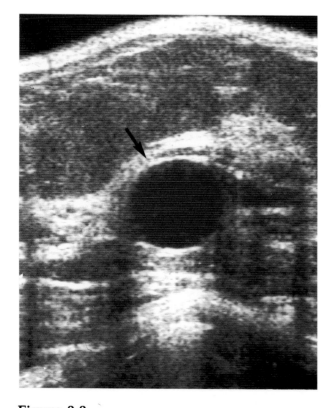

Figure 3.3

Breast sonography. Section through center of mass (arrow) shows typical findings of a cyst: anechoic interior, sharp anterior and posterior margins and enhancement of distal echoes.

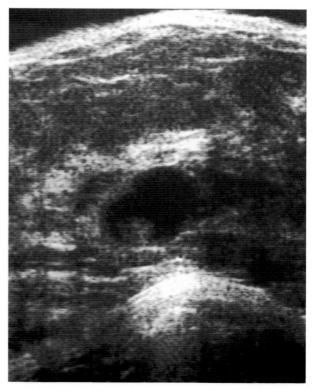

Figure 3.4

Breast sonography. In this section the cyst is lobulated. There appears to be a small nodule in the cyst wall.

Arterial calcifications are commonly seen in mammograms, particularly in the breasts of older women. The calcification is located in the wall of the vessel and results in tortuous, 'railroad track' parallel streaks of calcification following its course. Although it had been suggested that they are a sign of diabetes when they are found in the breasts of younger women, mammary arterial calcifications are now thought to have no clinical significance.[133]

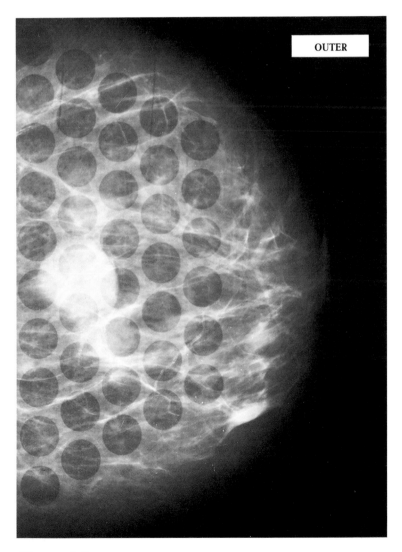

Figure 3.5

Cephalocaudal mammogram. The holes in the perforated compression plate are used to guide needle placement for pneumocystography.

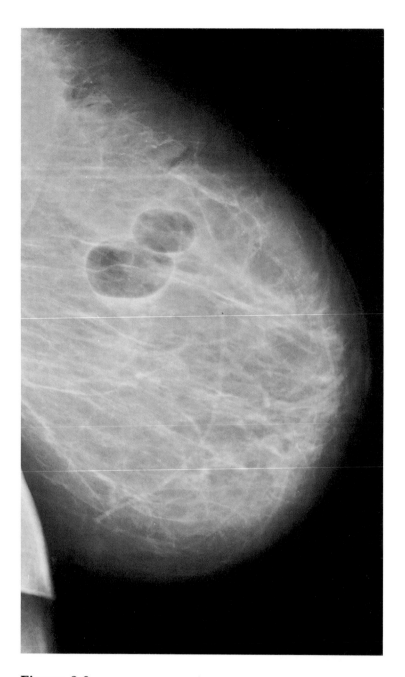

Figure 3.6

Pneumocystogram. Lining of the cyst is outlined with air and is smooth.

Case 4

This 54-year-old woman was asymptomatic.

Films: Right *(Figure 4.1)* and left *(Figure 4.2)* cephalocaudal mammograms.

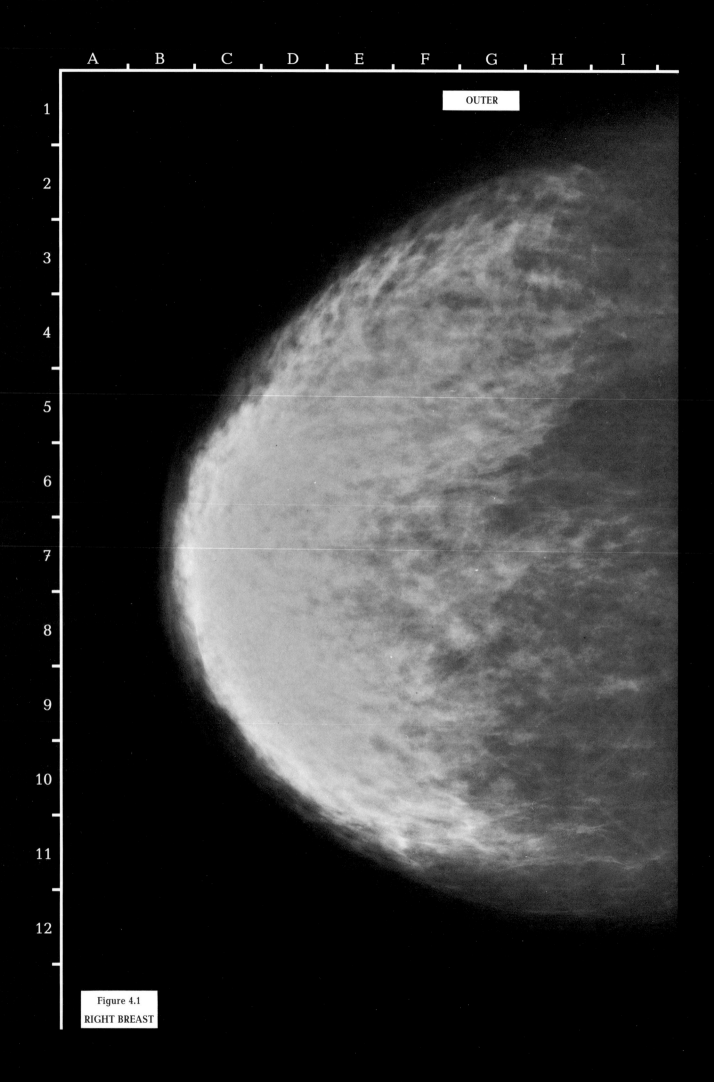

OUTER

Figure 4.1
RIGHT BREAST

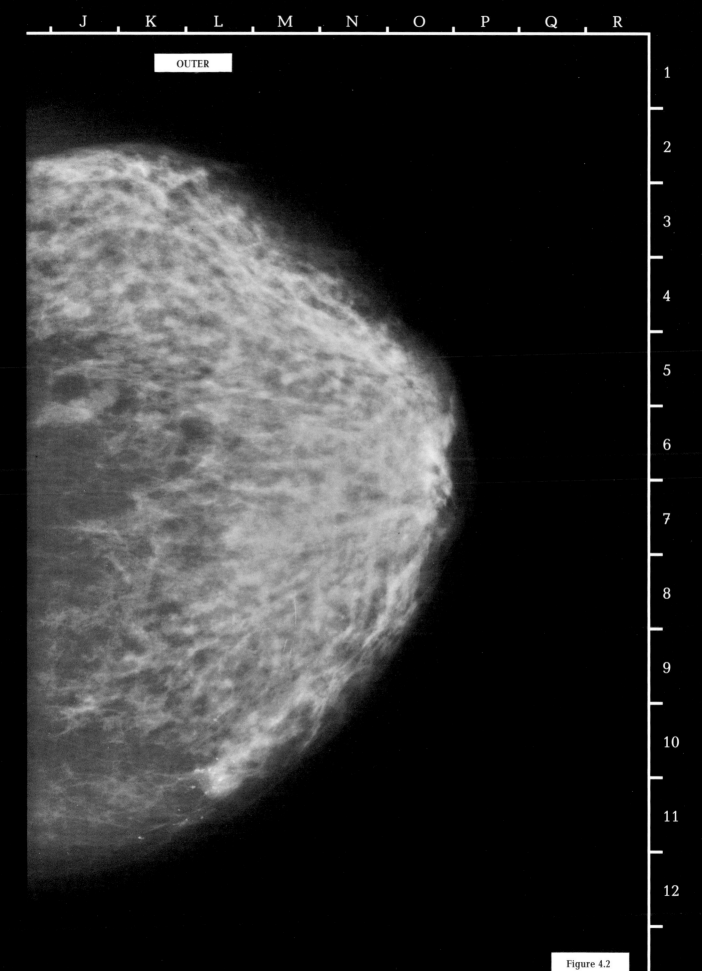

Figure 4.2
LEFT BREAST

Findings

The breasts are dense, showing a diffusely prominent ductal pattern bilaterally. There is a cluster of calcifications (L11) in the inner hemisphere of the left breast.

Discussion

The microcalcifications show features suspicious for malignancy: they are numerous, clustered, and of varying sizes and shapes *(Figure 4.3).*[83,143] A cluster can be defined as five or more discrete calcifications within $1\,cm^2$ of breast tissue.[129] Some of the calcifications appear as casts of the ducts, presenting elongate and branching patterns. Following needle localization, a biopsy was performed. A radiograph of the excised specimen verified that the nonpalpable suspicious area was removed *(Figure 4.4)*. Histologic examination showed infiltrating ductal carcinoma with coexisting intraductal carcinoma *(Figure 4.5)*. In the latter, calcification is present.

Calcifications may be the only sign of malignancy.[39,83,101,114] In a recent review of 300 nonpalpable cancers, calcifications were found to be the only sign of malignancy in 36 percent.[128]

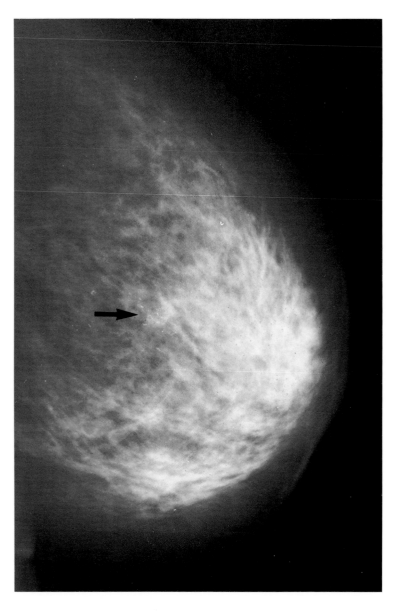

Figure 4.3

Mediolateral view shows the calcifications (arrow) in the upper hemisphere.

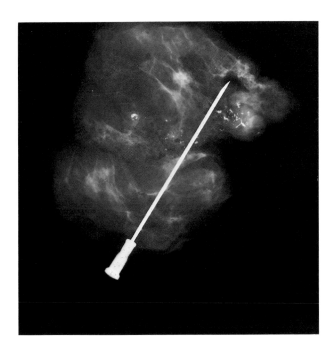

Figure 4.4

Specimen radiograph.

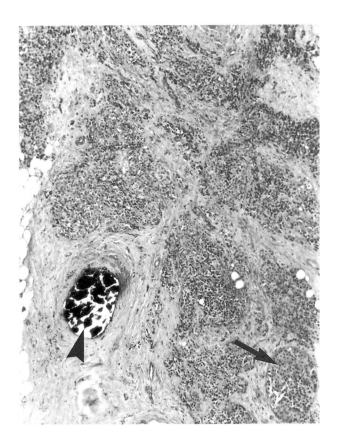

Figure 4.5

Low-power histologic section. Malignant cells widely infiltrate the breast tissue. Other tumor cells are confined to the preexisting duct (intraductal carcinoma) (arrow). Central necrosis and dystrophic calcification often occur in intraductal carcinoma (arrowhead). **Diagnosis**: Intraductal and infiltrating ductal carcinoma.

Case 5

This 56-year-old woman was referred for a screening mammogram.

Films: Right *(Figure 5.1)* and left *(Figure 5.2)* cephalocaudal views.

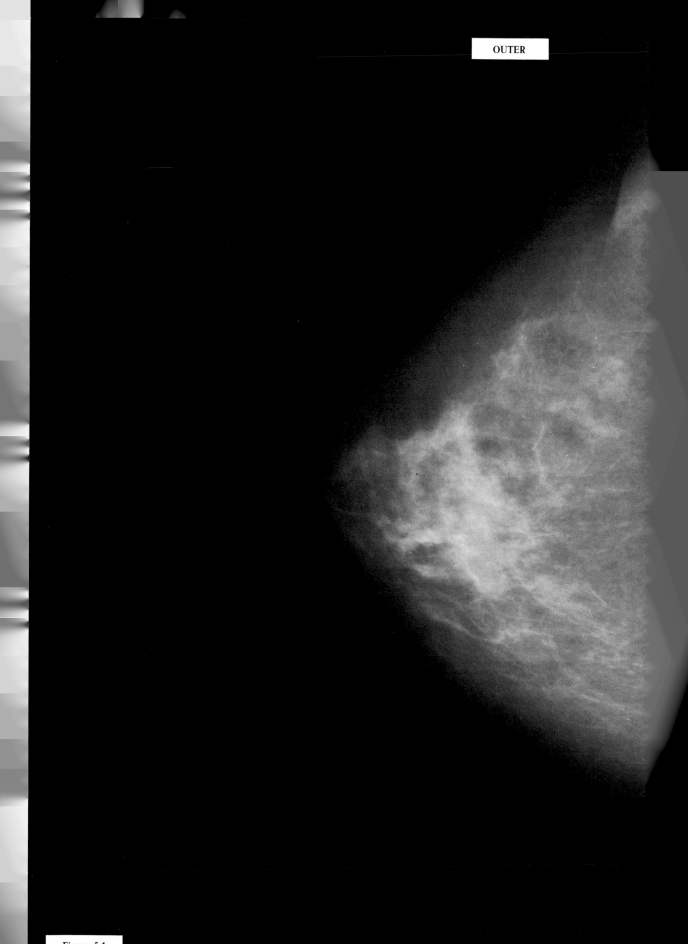

OUTER

Figure 5.1
RIGHT BREAST

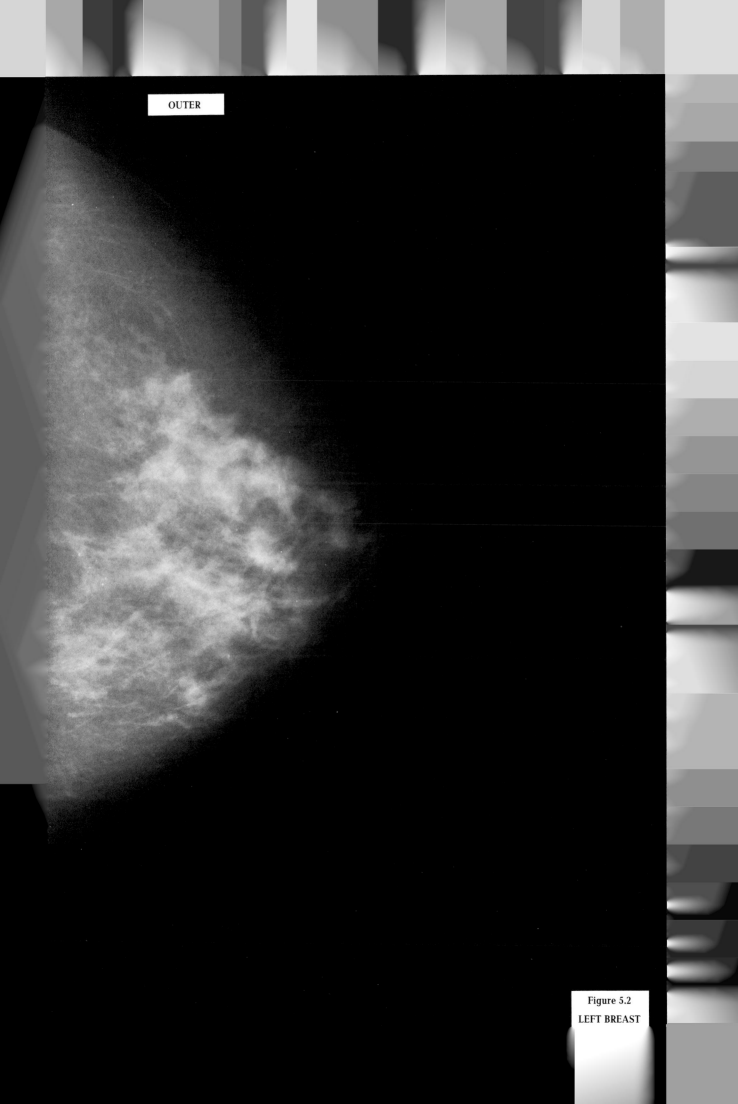

OUTER

Figure 5.2
LEFT BREAST

Findings

There is a cluster of microcalcifications deep in the left breast (J7).

Discussion

The calcifications are numerous and varying in size and shape. Their appearance is indetermin-ate, and carcinoma cannot be ruled out. Biopsy preceded by needle localization was recommended *(Figures 5.3 and 5.4)*. The specimen radiograph confirms that the calcifications were excised *(Figure 5.5)*. The biopsy revealed fibrocystic changes, including sclerosing adenosis *(Figure 5.6 and 5.7)*.

Clustered calcifications may be the only sign of malignancy.[127] However, benign conditions such as sclerosing adenosis and fat necrosis may result

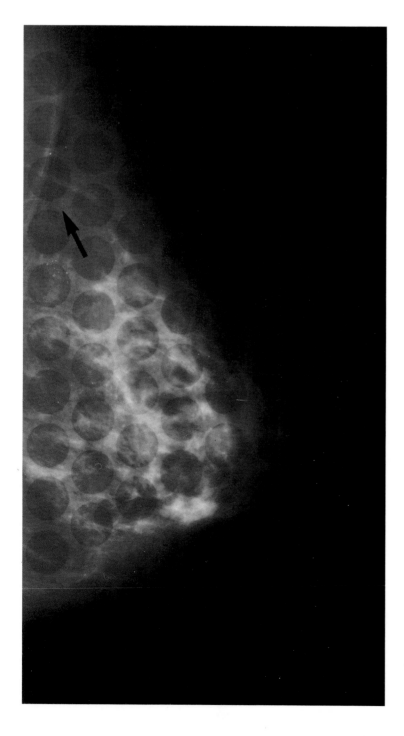

Figure 5.3

Mediolateral mammogram at time of prebiopsy needle localization. Compression was applied with a perforated hole plate. The localization needle will be placed through the hole directly overlying the calcifications (arrow).

in microcalcifications that mimic those of malignancy. In these benign disorders, the calcifications are usually more uniform, round, fewer in number and more scattered in distribution than the calcifications of malignancy. However, these signs are so nonspecific that most radiographically demonstrable clusters of stippled calcifications ultimately undergo histopathologic study.[39] Because they may be shattered or dislodged by the microtome blade during the preparation of the histologic sections, the calcifications seen in the mammogram cannot always be identified histologically.

Prebiopsy needle localization provides an accurate method for biopsy of these calcifications with minimal subsequent deformity.[146] The use of a compression plate modified for localization procedures and a grid-coordinate system expedites the placement of the needle tip at the site of a nonpalpable lesion.[65,67,74,75] Once the needle is in position, a barbed tip or J-hookwire can be

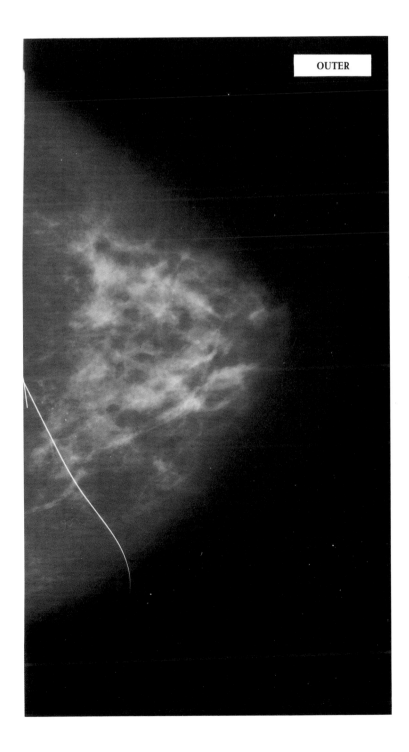

OUTER

Figure 5.4

Cephalocaudal mammogram shows hookwire at site of calcifications.

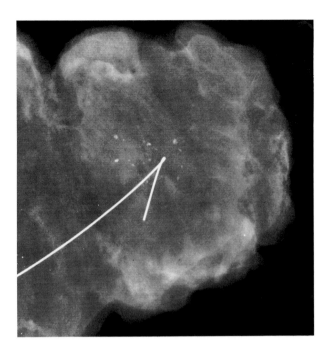

afterloaded through the needle. Once the specimen is excised it is essential to perform a radiograph of the specimen to ensure that the calcifications have been included.[63,139]

Figure 5.5

Specimen radiograph verifies that the calcifications have been removed.

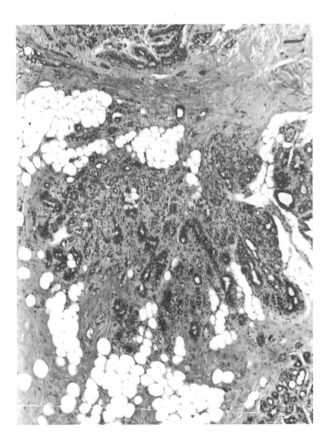

Figure 5.6

Low-power histologic section. A proliferation of terminal ducts and lobules takes the form of nests and cords of cells within a fibrous stroma. **Diagnosis**: sclerosing adenosis.

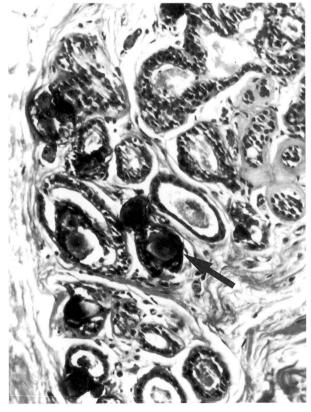

Figure 5.7

High-power histologic section. Microcalcifications (arrow) are seen within the acini.

Case 6

This 28-year-old woman who had discontinued breastfeeding her baby 6 months earlier complained of right breast tenderness.

Films: Mediolateral oblique *(Figure 6.1)* and cephalocaudal *(Figure 6.2)* views of the right breast.

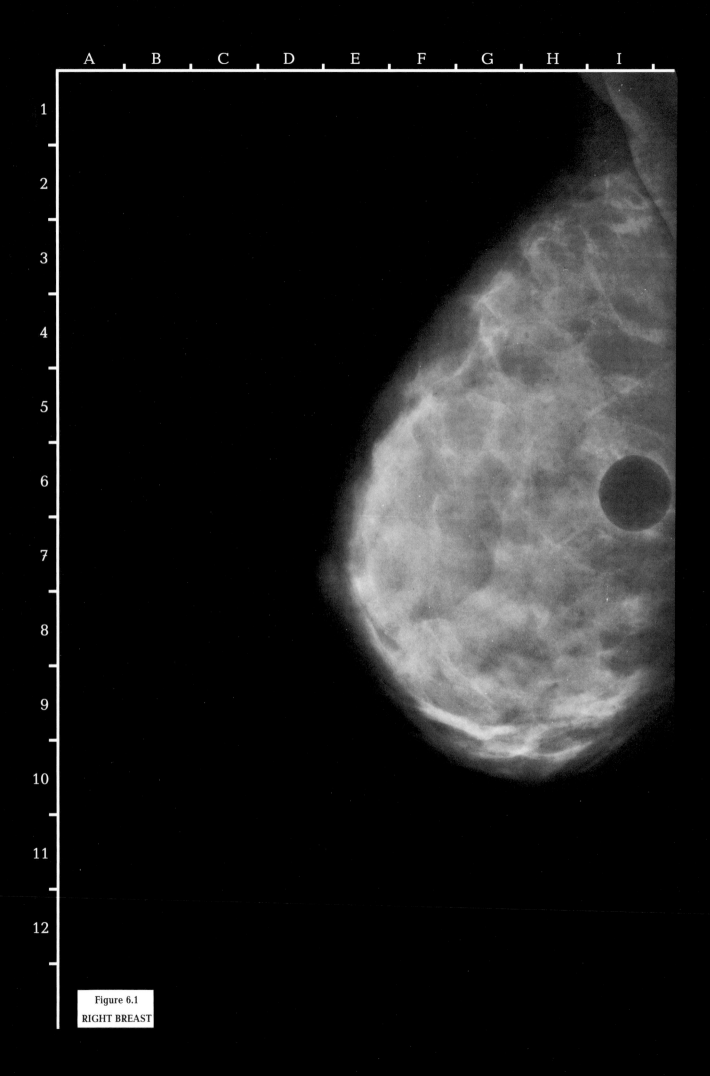

Figure 6.1
RIGHT BREAST

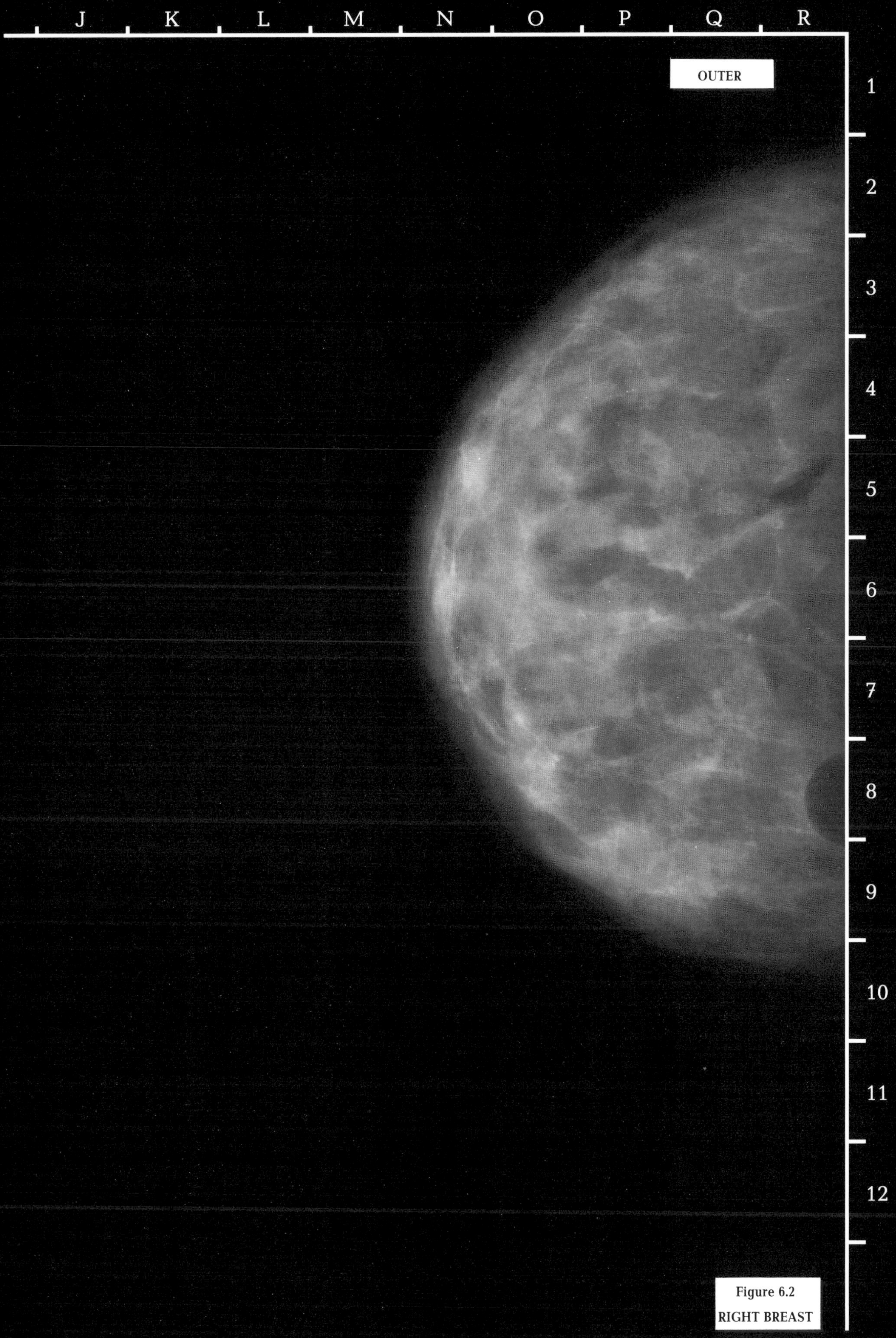

J K L M N O P Q R

OUTER

1
2
3
4
5
6
7
8
9
10
11
12

Figure 6.2
RIGHT BREAST

Findings

There is a sharply outlined round radiolucency in the upper–inner quadrant of the right breast seen in both oblique (I6) and cephalocaudal views (R8).

Discussion

The history of recent breast feeding is the important factor in the diagnosis. The radiographic features are consistent with a galactocele. Galactoceles are benign breast cysts that contain milk[54] and, when palpable, are freely movable. They usually occur 6–10 months after the cessation of lactation. The lactiferous material in the galactocele is responsible for the radiolucency, and the round shape is the result of compression on this fluid-filled structure. Galactoceles may also have mixed density and a fat-water level.[31] Occasionally it may be useful to aspirate a palpable galactocele. The aspiration will yield characteristic milky fluid and the mass will disappear. In this case, the galactocele was an incidental finding, and the tenderness resolved without any intervention.

Lipomas and post-traumatic oil cysts are other radiolucent masses that may be observed in mammograms. Lipomas are more often oval than perfectly round and they have a delicate capsule which is visible in mammograms. Usually, they are nonpalpable and solitary. They are easier to identify when the surrounding breast tissue is dense. Occasionally they have central calcification, indicating infarction.[31] Lipomas are more likely to be found in the breasts of older than younger women, with a reported average age of 47 years.[54] A post-traumatic oil cyst is more likely to occur in the periareolar area where blunt trauma is more common or at the site of previous surgery. Oil cysts have a fibrous capsule that may contain calcification, and fat necrosis may be manifested by additional radiographic findings such as architectural distortion and skin thickening.[14]

Case 7

This 74-year-old woman was asymptomatic.

Films: Mediolateral oblique view of right *(Figure 7.1)* and left *(Figure 7.2)* breasts.

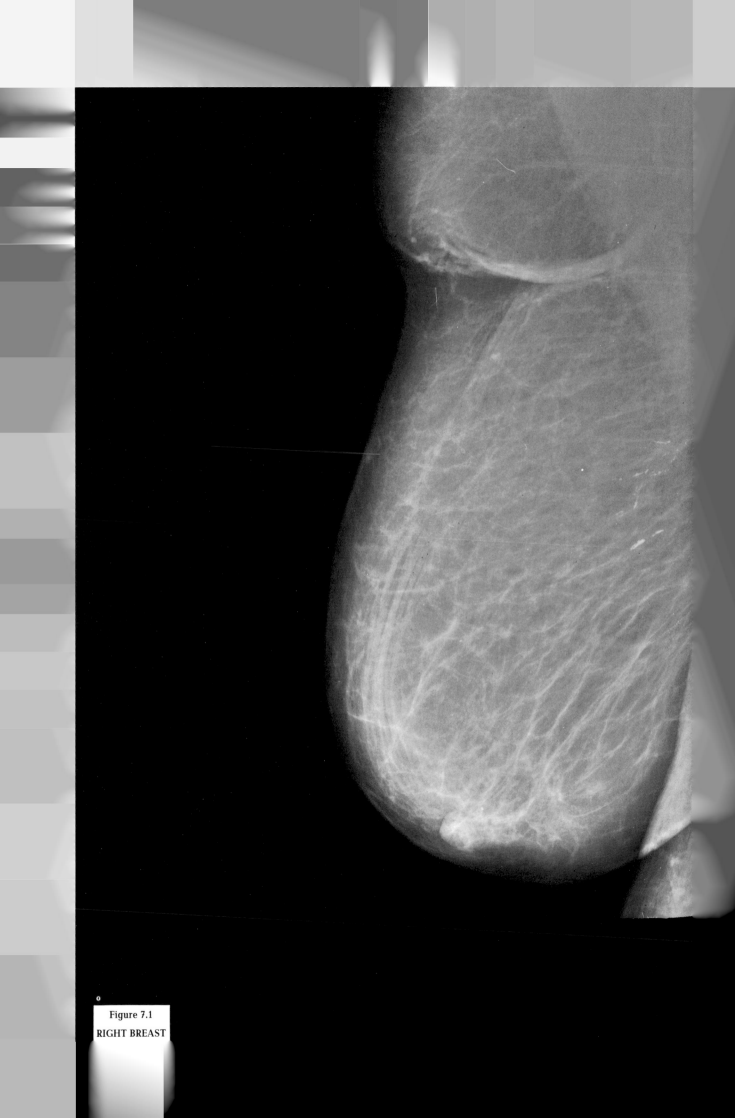

Figure 7.1
RIGHT BREAST

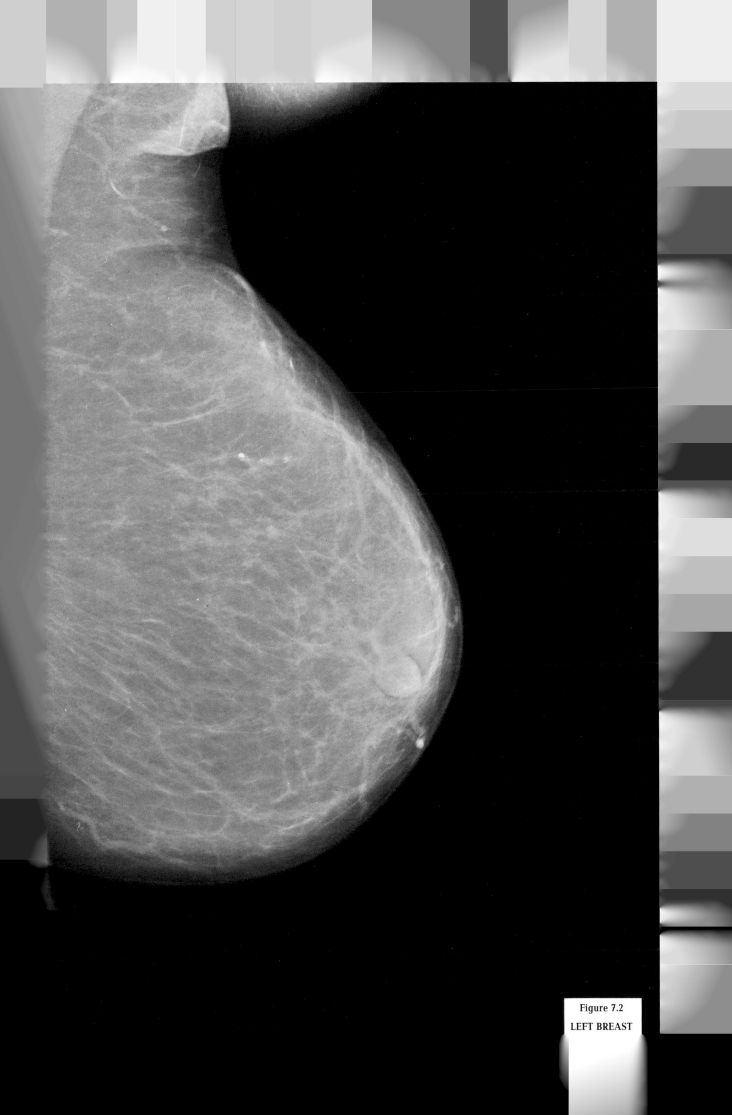

Figure 7.2
LEFT BREAST

Findings

The breasts are fatty. There are clusters of micro-calcifications in both the right (I6) and left (M6) breasts, as well as vascular calcifications in the left breast (J9). Several skin folds (E8) result from mammographic compression of the atrophied breasts.

Discussion

The calcifications in the right breast are irregular in contour, linear and branching, reflecting the shapes of the ducts *(Figure 7.3)*. These casting calcifications are said to be characteristic of carcinoma.[143] The calcifications in the left breast are also irregular in shape and of various sizes *(Figure 7.4)*. Biopsy would be the only way to be certain of their etiology. Following bilateral mammographically guided needle localizations, biopsies were performed. The histologic examination of the right breast biopsy specimen revealed intraductal and infiltrating ductal carcinoma *(Figures 7.5 and 7.6)*. The calcifications in the left breast were due to fibrocystic changes.

Malignant intraductal calcifications typically appear fragmented and have irregular shapes and varying sizes. Casting calcifications are said to be

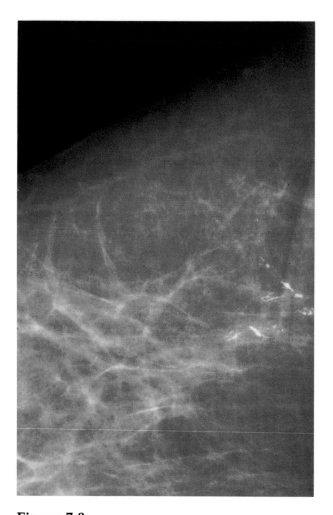

Figure 7.3

Close-up of right breast calcifications.

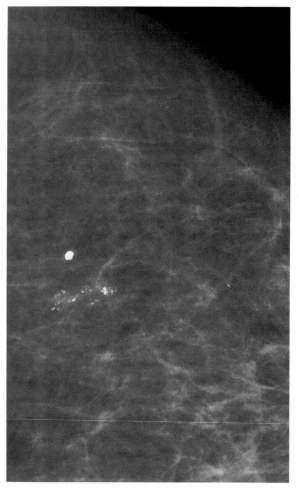

Figure 7.4

Close-up of left breast calcifications.

the most reliable sign of intraductal carcinoma. These calcifications, casts of the duct lumens, have linear and branching patterns, representing necrosis of malignant cells within the ducts *(Figures 7.5 and 7.6)*.

The origin of the calcifications in benign conditions is not known. However, it has been hypothesized that they may be secondary to active secretion or chemical changes in the tissues.[85]

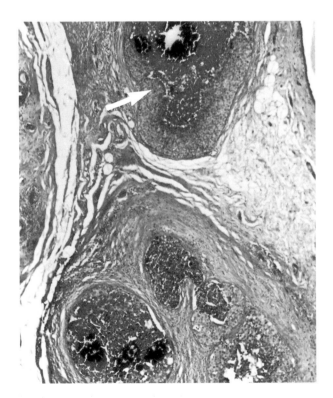

Figure 7.5

Low-power histologic section of right breast specimen. The intraductal carcinoma is characterized by ducts which are dilated and filled with neoplastic epithelial cells that completely plug the lumens (arrow). Central necrosis and calcification are typical of the comedo variant of intraductal carcinoma. Periductal fibrosis is prominent. Elsewhere there is infiltrating ductal carcinoma which is not demonstrated here. **Diagnosis**: Intraductal and infiltrating ductal carcinoma.

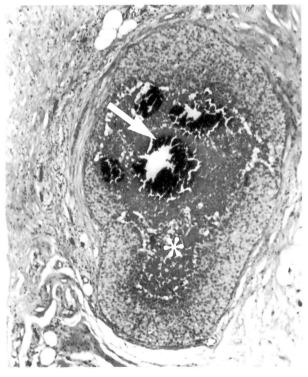

Figure 7.6

High-power histologic section of right breast specimen. Central areas of necrotic tumor cells (asterisk) and dystrophic calcification (arrow) are evident within the duct.

Case 8

This 53-year-old woman had a right mastectomy and a biopsy of the left breast 7 years ago. She was referred for a routine mammogram of the left breast.

Films: Mediolateral view of the left breast *(Figure 8.1).*

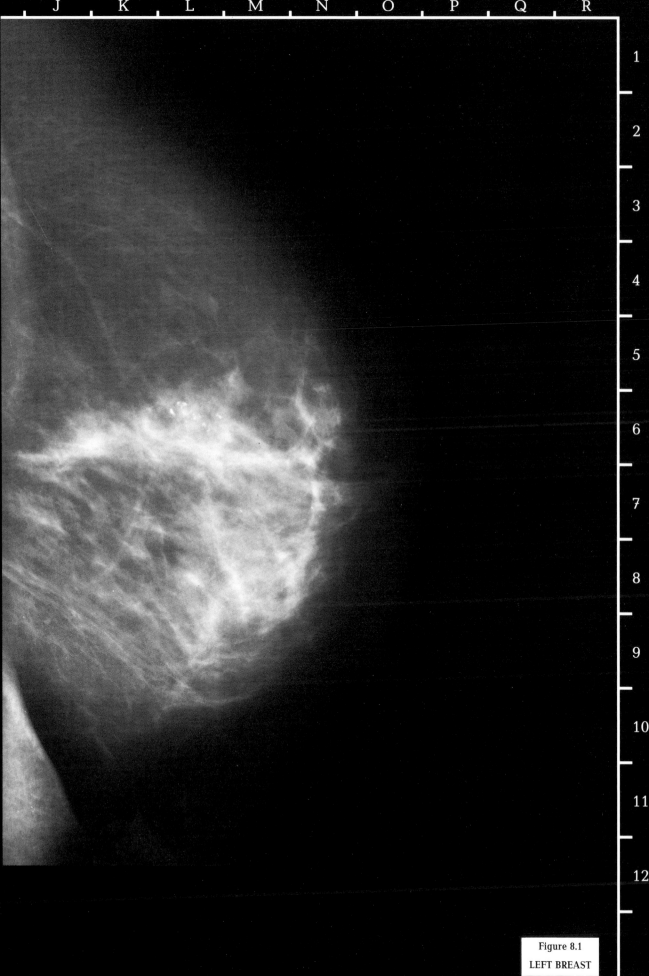

Figure 8.1
LEFT BREAST

Findings

There is a cluster of calcifications (L6). The calcifications overlie two cyst-like areas of fat density.

Discussion

The lipid-density (oil) cysts were also seen in the cephalocaudal mammogram *(Figure 8.2)*. The calcifications are mildly suspicious for malignancy, but the presence of the lipid-density cysts and the history of a previous biopsy suggest post-traumatic fat necrosis. Although the mammographic diagnosis was benign fat necrosis, a biopsy was performed because of the patient's history of contralateral breast carcinoma and the indeterminate appearance of the calcifications. Histologic diagnosis was fat necrosis *(Figure 8.3)*.

Traumatic fat necrosis of the breast is a nonsuppurative inflammatory process which may result in any one of a variety of radiographic appearances, some of which may be confused with carcinoma.[2] The spectrum of mammographic features of fat necrosis includes a spiculated density; localized

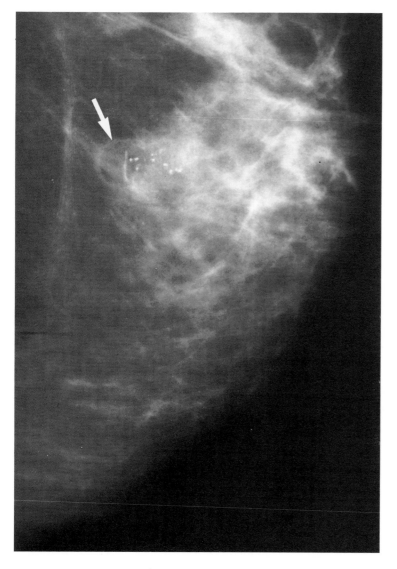

Figure 8.2

Cephalocaudal projection. A lipid-density cyst (arrow) is clearly visualized.

thickening and deformity of the skin; branching, rod-like or angular microcalcifications, and lipid-filled cysts with or without calcified walls.[14,15]

Clinically, fat necrosis may be asymptomatic and without abnormal physical findings, or it may result in an indurated mass. It is characteristically situated near the skin or areola, since these are the sites within the breast that are most vulnerable to trauma, especially that of surgery. The palpable mass may enlarge slowly over a period of weeks and may or may not undergo spontaneous regression. Although blunt trauma may result in fat necrosis, prior surgery is the most frequent cause.

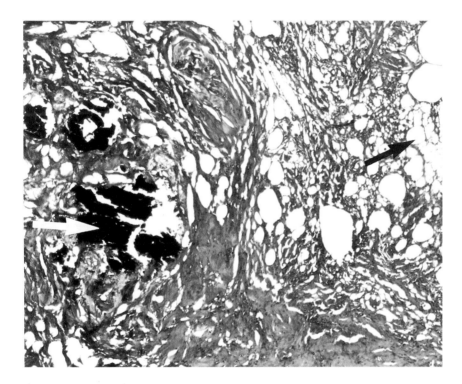

Figure 8.3

High-power histologic section. There are multiple, irregularly sized, lipid-filled cysts (black arrow) surrounded by dense fibrosis. Calcifications (white arrow) are found within several of the cysts. **Diagnosis**: Fat necrosis.

Case 9

A 57-year-old woman felt a soft lump near the nipple of her right breast.

Films: Right *(Figure 9.1)* and left *(Figure 9.2)* mediolateral views.

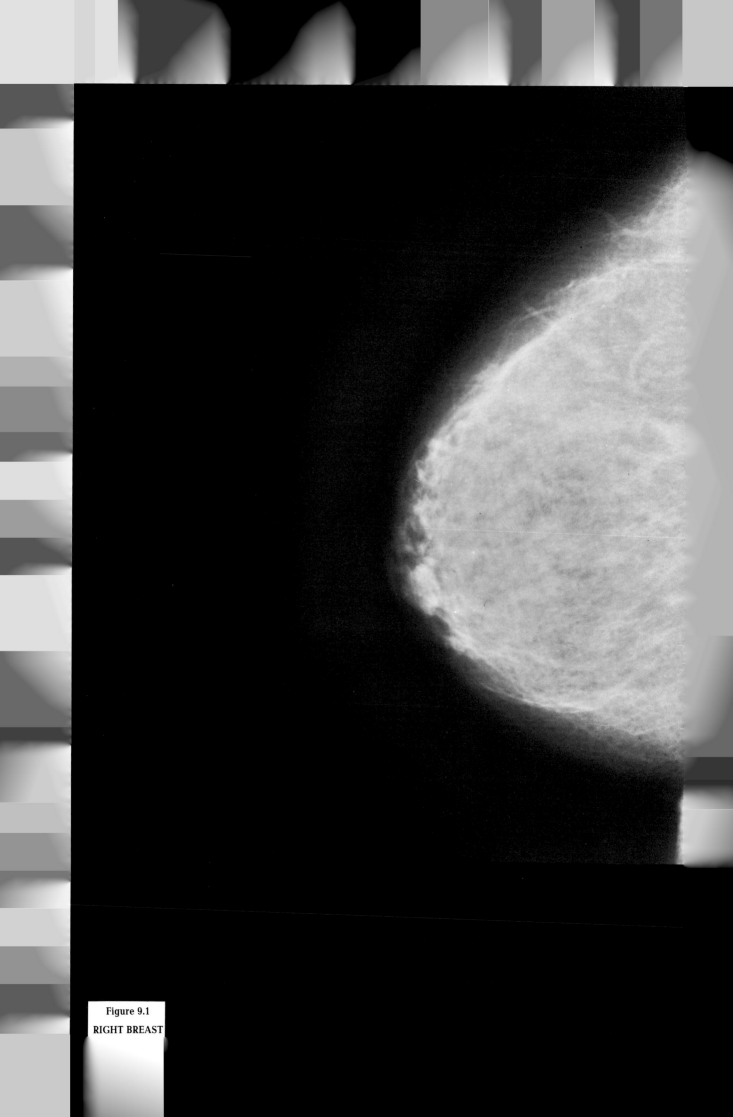

Figure 9.1
RIGHT BREAST

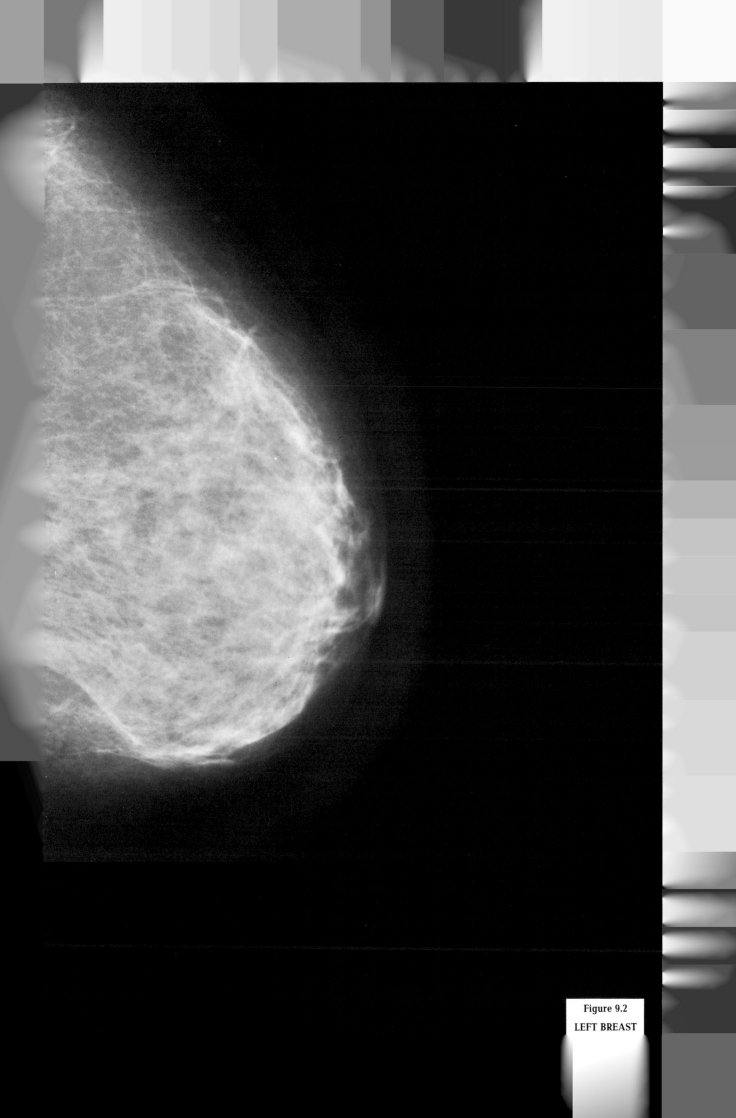

Figure 9.2
LEFT BREAST

Findings

There is a 1 cm mass (F7) in the right breast. There are also a few isolated benign calcifications.

Discussion

The right subareolar mass is lobulated, well circumscribed, and of intermediate radiographic density. In a younger woman, these mammographic features would suggest a benign mass such as fibroadenoma. However, in a woman aged 57, a well-circumscribed carcinoma must be excluded. Because the mass was soft at palpation, a cyst was also considered in the differential diagnosis. Because needle aspiration failed to yield fluid, an open biopsy was performed. Histologic diagnosis was mucinous (colloid) carcinoma.

Invasive duct carcinoma typically has irregular margins indicative of its infiltrative nature. However, some breast cancers have margins that are smooth, mimicking a benign lesion,[153] and these well-defined tumors have a better prognosis overall.[81] Examples of breast cancers that are more likely to have well-demarcated margins are medullary, colloid and papillary carcinomas. However, the majority of carcinomas with rounded, well-delimited margins are duct carcinomas of not otherwise specified type, which are the most common histologic type of breast carcinoma.[81] Since carcinomas may present with well-defined margins, open or needle biopsy should be performed for any palpable solid mass, and a biopsy should be considered for any dominant mammographically detected solid mass. A dominant mass is one that is solitary and over 5 mm in diameter, one that stands out from other masses, one with suspicious radiographic features (irregular margins, associated clustered calcifications), one that is enlarging on serial mammogram or one that is not present on previous mammograms.

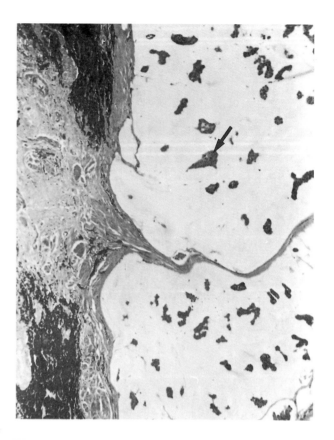

Figure 9.3

Low-power histologic specimen. There are lakes of amorphous lightly staining mucin extending into surrounding tissue. The fibrous capsule around the tumor is distended by the fluid-filled contents, and causes the well-circumscribed margin seen in the mammogram. Small islands of neoplastic cells (arrow) are seen within the mucinous pool. **Diagnosis**: Mucinous (colloid) carcinoma.

Mucinous carcinomas tend to grow slowly, and have favorable outcome, but if not treated they eventually metastasize to the axillary lymph nodes and beyond.[25] They may be well delineated and soft to palpation and thus mistaken for a benign cyst.[54] In these tumors, mucin secreted by the carcinoma cells accumulates in large amounts.

Case 10

This 63-year-old woman reported a right breast mass. The mass could not be palpated at the time of mammography.

Films: Right *(Figure 10.1)* and left *(Figure 10.2)* mediolateral mammograms.

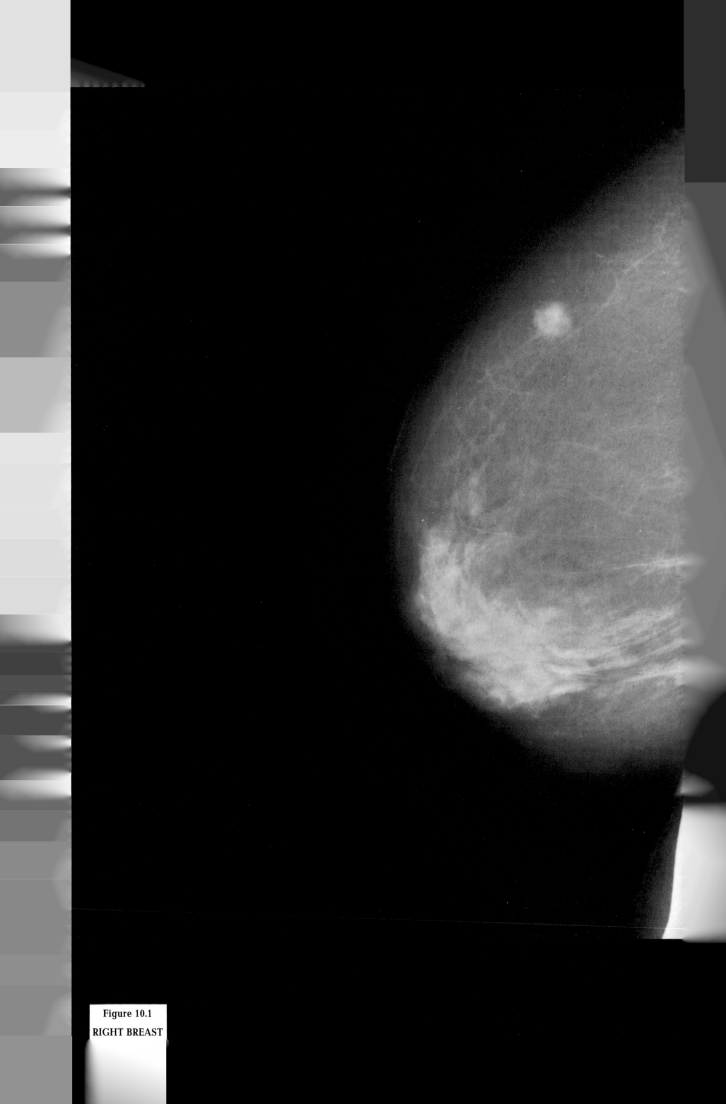

Figure 10.1
RIGHT BREAST

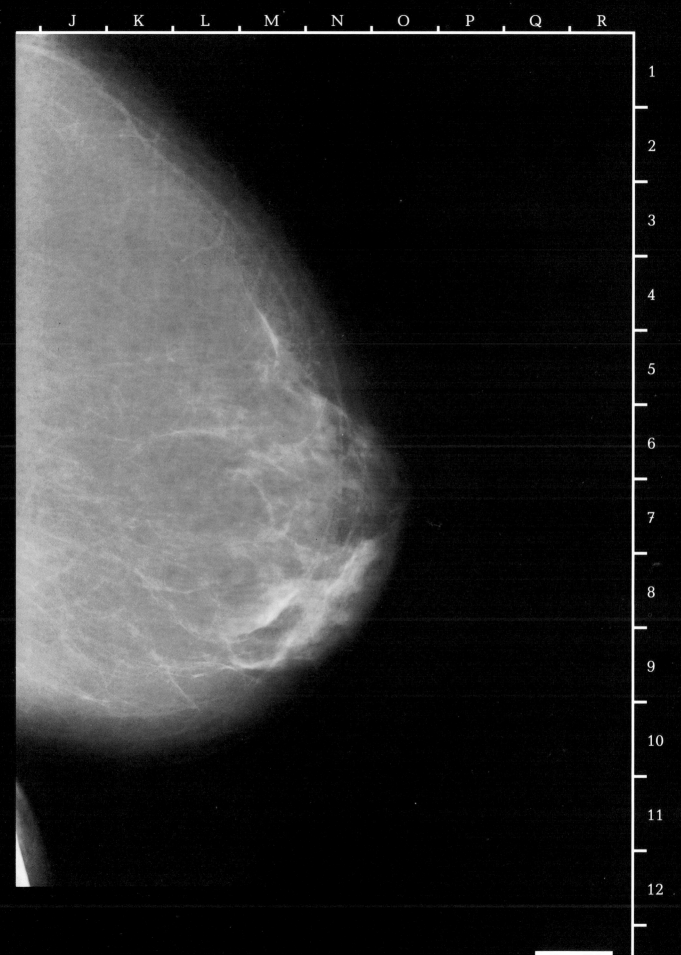

Figure 10.2
LEFT BREAST

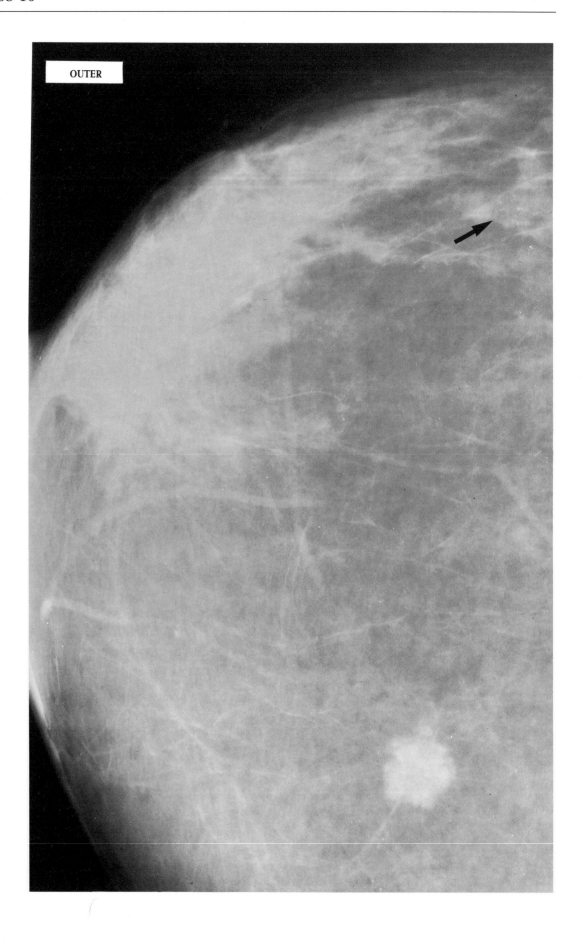

Findings

There is a lobulated 1 cm mass (H4) in the upper hemisphere of the right breast. Clusters of calcifications are barely visible in the right breast within the dense subareolar tissue (I8). The left breast is larger, but it is otherwise unremarkable.

Discussion

A magnification cephalocaudal view confirms the irregular margins of the right breast mass *(Figure 10.3)*. In the magnification film, the calcifications in the outer hemisphere are shown to be numerous and clustered. Biopsy of the mass and the calcifications revealed that both represented foci of carcinoma.

Breast cancer has been reported to be mammographically multifocal or multicentric at the time of mammographic detection in 15 percent of cases.[128] Multifocal carcinoma can be defined as two foci separated by at least 20 mm of benign tissue. Multicentric carcinoma indicates cancer in two different quadrants, and includes concomitant bilateral carcinoma.[97] Mammographic detection of multicentric carcinoma is important since many surgeons and radiation oncologists feel that it is a contraindication to breast-conserving treatment. Multifocal carcinoma may be suitable for local resection and radiotherapy, but it is important that all of the tumor is removed prior to radiotherapy and that this is confirmed histologically by identification of tumor-free margins in the operative specimen.

Figure 10.3

Magnification cephalocaudal mammogram shows the irregularly marginated mass and the microcalcifications (arrow). **Pathologic diagnosis**: multicentric carcinoma.

Case 11

This 43-year-old woman complained of a 'tugging' sensation under the nipple of her left breast.

Films: Right *(Figure 11.1)* and left *(Figure 11.2)* mediolateral oblique mammograms, and right *(Figure 11.3)* and left *(Figure 11.4)* cephalocaudal mammograms.

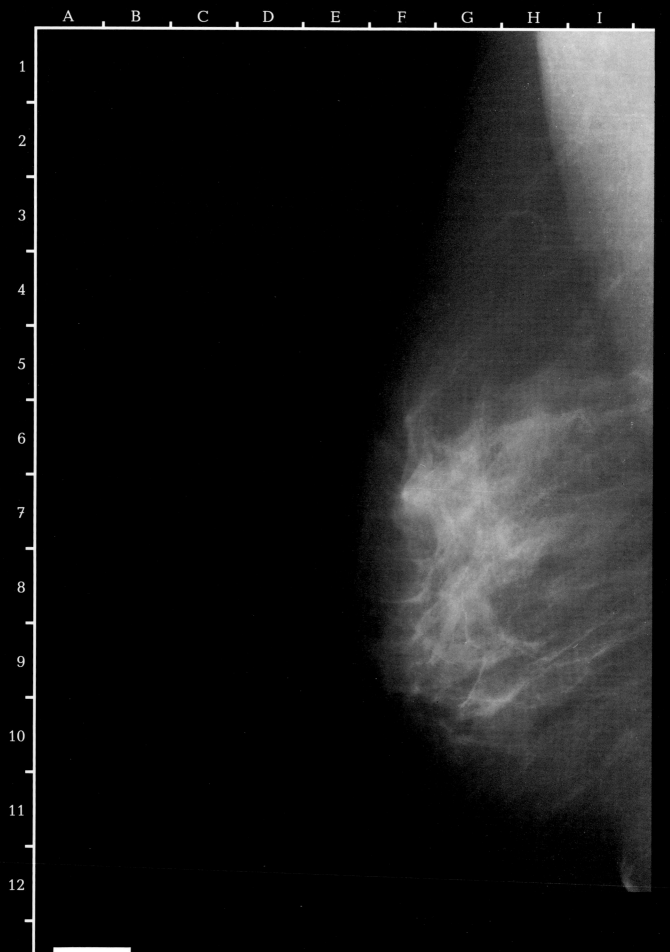

Figure 11.1
RIGHT BREAST

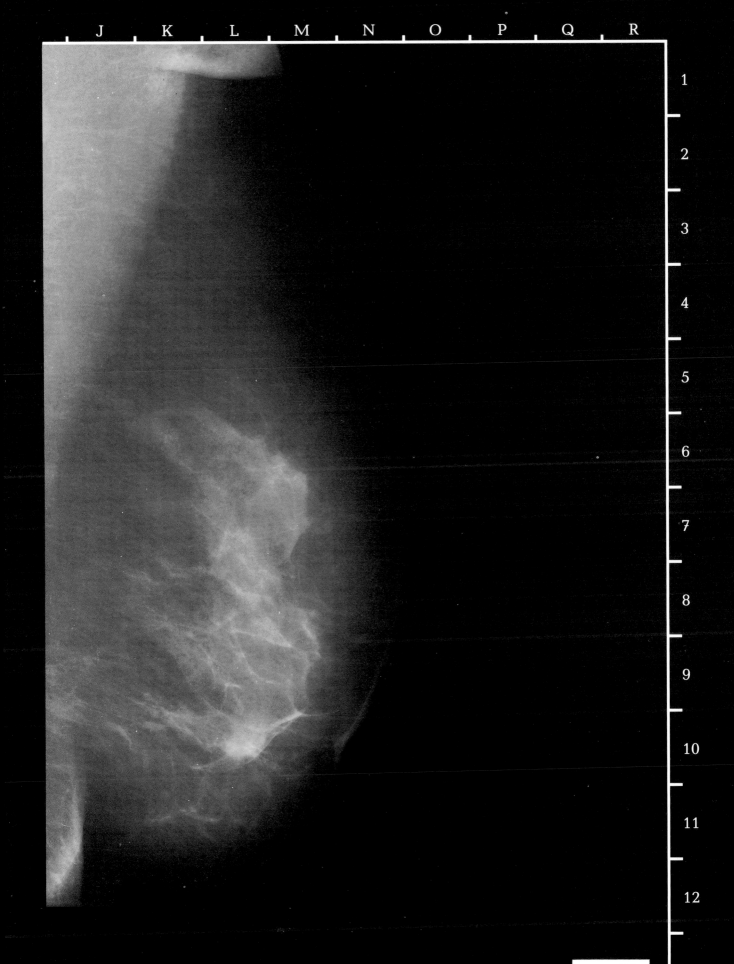

J K L M N O P Q R

1

2

3

4

5

6

7

8

9

10

11

12

Figure 11.2
LEFT BREAST

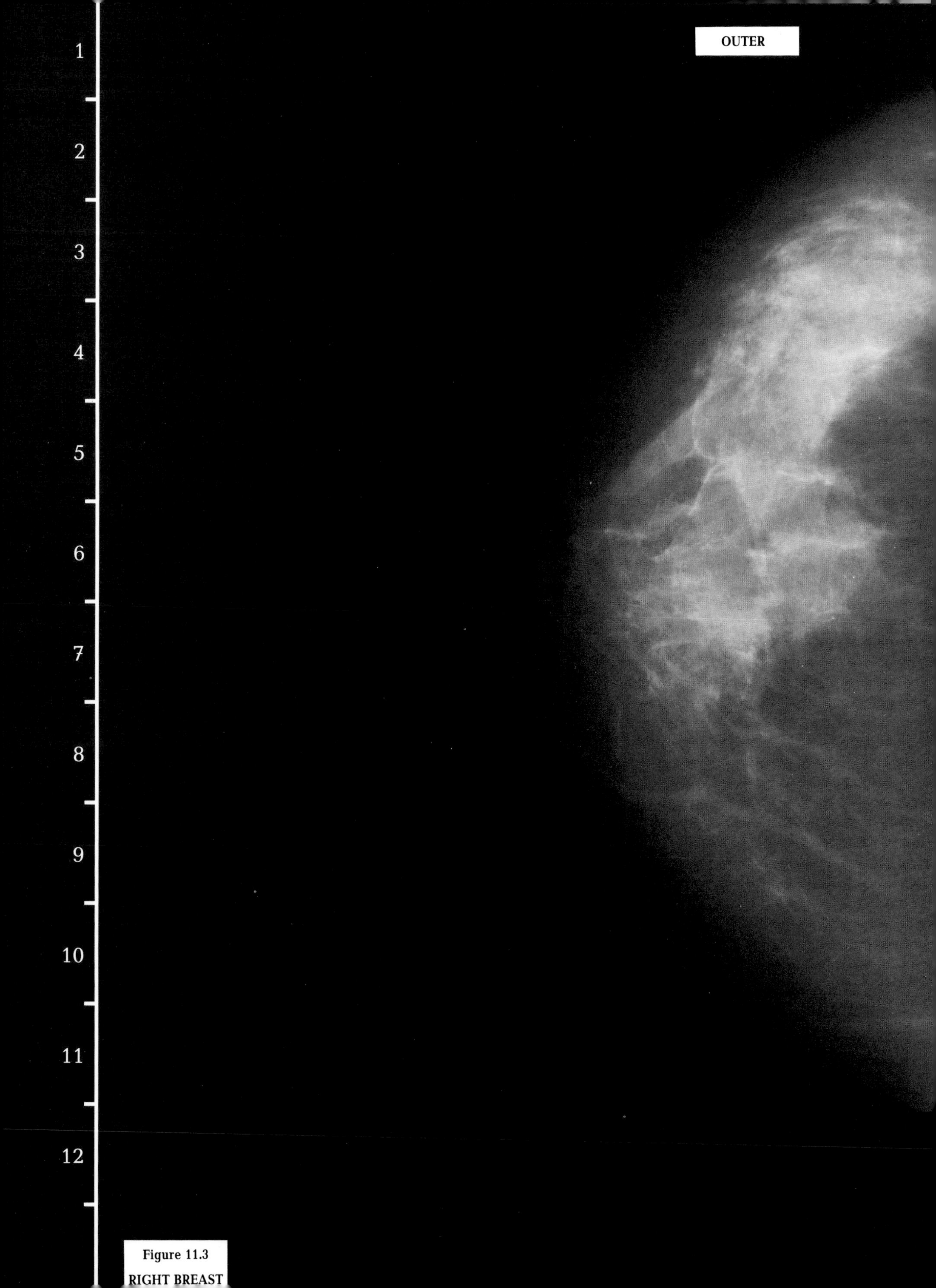

OUTER

1
2
3
4
5
6
7
8
9
10
11
12

Figure 11.3
RIGHT BREAST

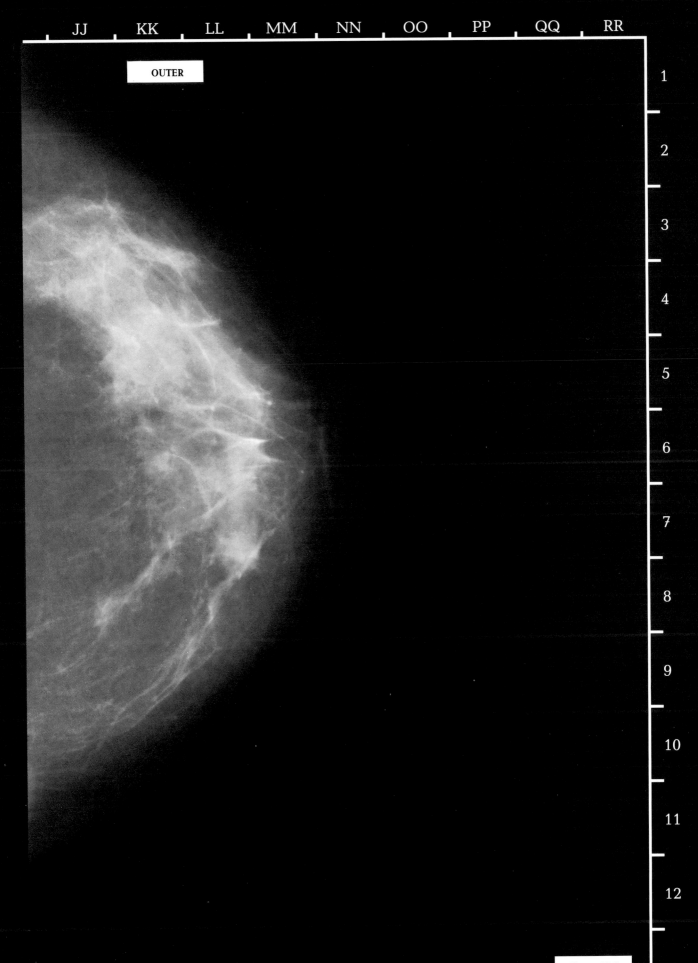

JJ KK LL MM NN OO PP QQ RR

OUTER

1
2
3
4
5
6
7
8
9
10
11
12

Figure 11.4
LEFT BREAST

Findings

There is an asymmetric, irregular 1 cm density in the subareolar region of the left breast (L10),(LL7). In addition, in the oblique projection there is a suggestion of skin retraction anterior to the mass (M10).

Discussion

The mass in the subareolar region of the left breast has two mammographic features suspicious of malignancy: irregular margins and high density compared to the surrounding parenchyma. There were no palpable abnormalities at the site of this mammographic abnormality, and nipple retraction was not evident on clinical examination but skin retraction was present on the oblique projection. Biopsy of the subareolar mass revealed infiltrating lobular carcinoma *(Figure 11.5)*.

Lobular carcinomas are believed to arise from the lobules and terminal ducts. Due to the variation in histologic criteria, their frequency varies from as high as 20 percent to as low as 1 percent.[34] They are bilateral in about 20 percent of cases,[149] a rate of bilaterality that is more frequent than for ductal carcinomas.[35] Lobular carcinoma also manifests a two-fold greater incidence of multicentricity in the same breast.[84] However, the overall survival rate for invasive lobular carcinoma is believed to be slightly better than for invasive ductal carcinoma.[34]

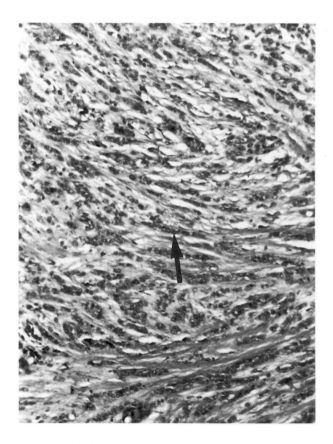

Figure 11.5

High-power histologic section. Infiltrating lobular carcinoma characterized by single files of cells (indian files) (arrow) and marked stromal desmoplastic response.

Case 12

This 47-year-old woman had an aspiration of a cyst in the left breast the day before these mammograms were performed. The mammograms were requested to 'rule out a right breast mass.' The left breast was red and tender in the periareolar area where multiple cyst punctures had been performed.

Films: Mediolateral views of the right *(Figure 12.1)* and left *(Figure 12.2)* breasts.

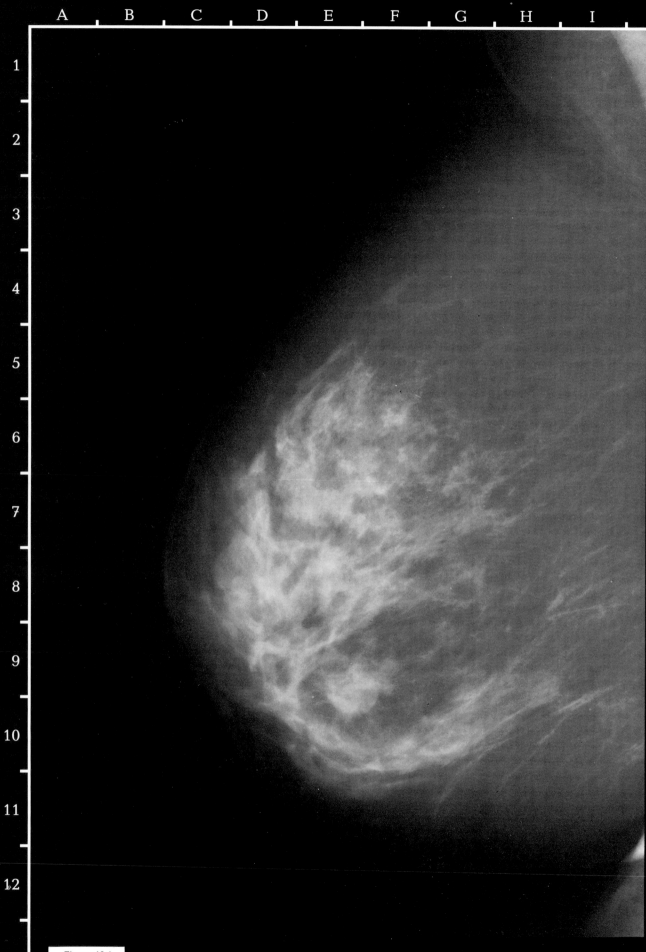

Figure 12.1
RIGHT BREAST

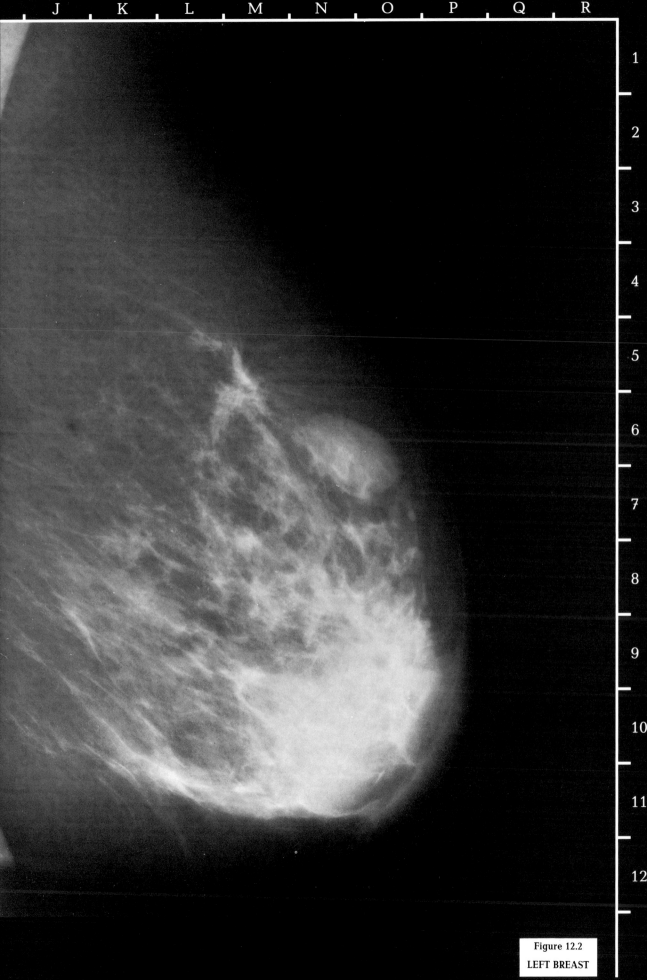

Figure 12.2
LEFT BREAST

Findings

There is a well-defined 12 mm mass in the right breast (E9).

In the left breast, there is increased density in the subareolar area and thickening of the overlying skin. A well-defined 3 cm oval mass is present (N6), and, posteriorly, a spiculated mass which contains faint microcalcifications (M5).

Discussion

The cephalocaudal view of the left breast (Figure 12.3) shows that the oval mass is directly posterior to the nipple. The spiculated lesion, highly suspicious for carcinoma, is directly posterior to the oval mass. Breast sonography revealed that the well-circumscribed 12 mm mass in the right breast and the larger well-circumscribed mass in the left breast were simple cysts. Biopsy was recommended for the spiculated mass, and revealed infiltrating ductal carcinoma.

This case illustrates the importance of mammography, even when a palpable mass yields cyst fluid. The carcinoma was located directly posterior to the cyst, and might have gone undetected, had not the mammograms been performed.

Cyst aspiration prior to mammography may lead to difficulties in performance and interpretation of the mammographic examination. If the aspiration is performed within a week of the mammogram, a resultant hematoma or edema can either mimic a malignant mass or cause a preexisting well-defined benign mass to have irregular and ill-defined margins, resulting in a false diagnosis of malignancy.[71]

In this patient, mammographic compression of the left breast was difficult due to pain and tenderness from multiple cyst aspirations. The cyst aspirations resulted in edema in the skin and subareolar tissues, making interpretation of the mammograms difficult.

These problems are not encountered when mammograms are delayed at least 2 weeks following needle aspiration. Clinicians should be encouraged to request mammography prior to needle aspiration, or to defer mammography for at least 2 weeks after needle aspiration.[135]

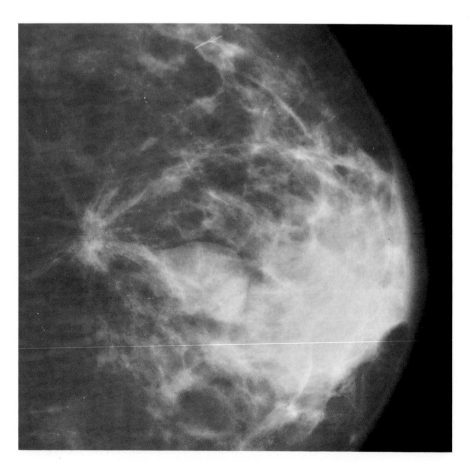

Figure 12.3

Close-up of left breast masses. The spiculated mass contains microcalcifications. **Pathologic diagnosis**: Infiltrating ductal carcinoma.

Case 13

This 69-year-old woman was referred for an abnormal mammogram of the left breast. Four months previously she had a biopsy of the left subareolar area, which was interpreted as lobular carcinoma in situ.

Films: Left mediolateral *(Figure 13.1)* and left cephalocaudal *(Figure 13.2)* mammograms.

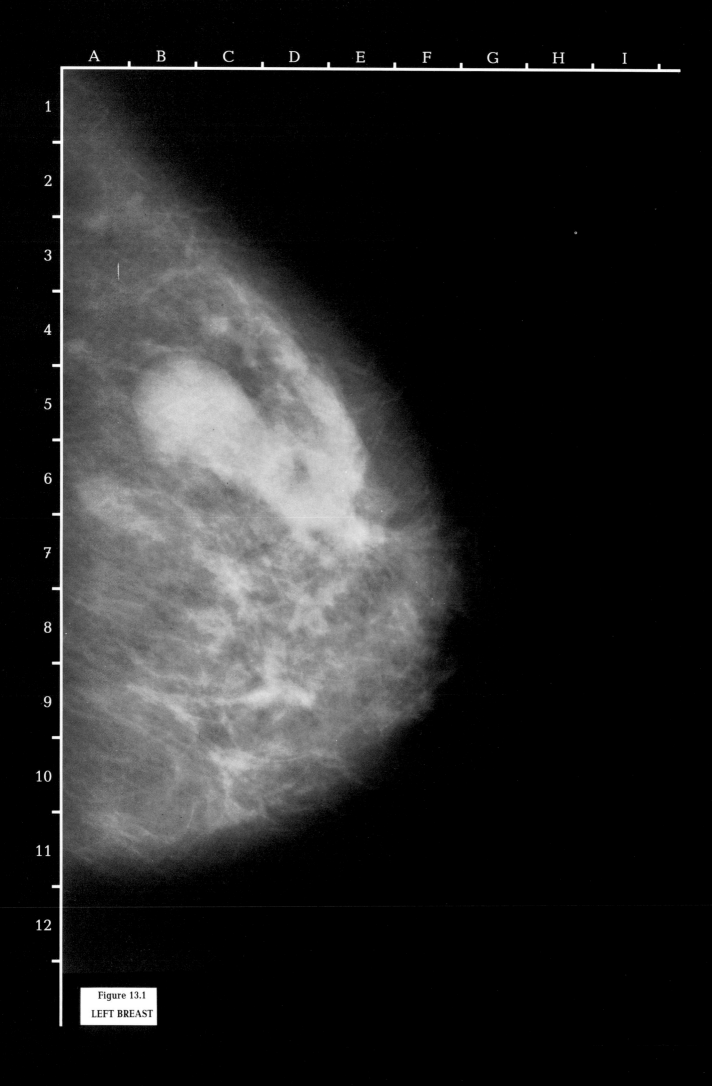

Figure 13.1
LEFT BREAST

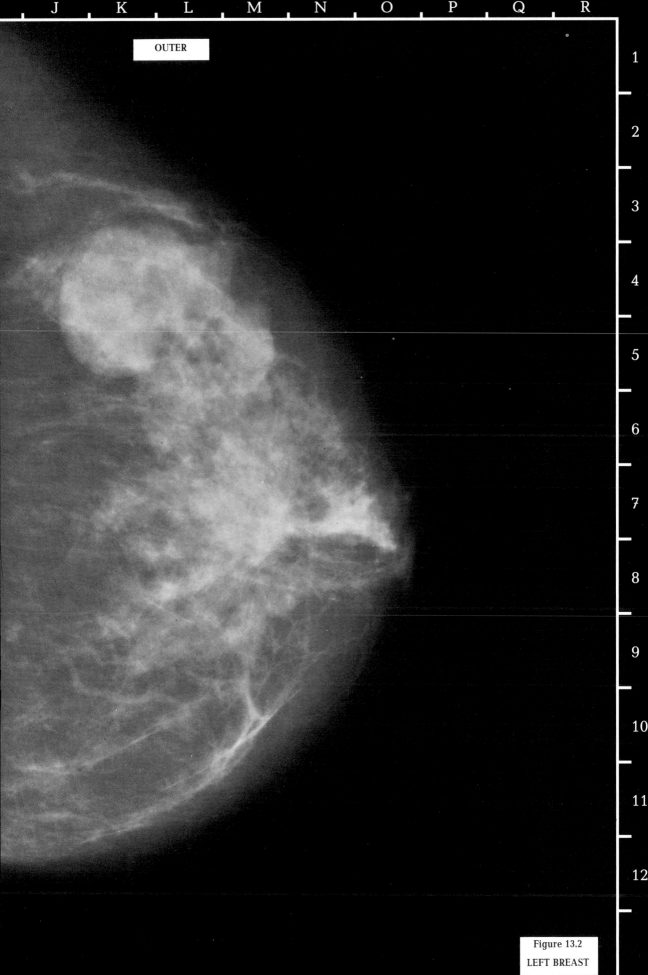

OUTER

Figure 13.2
LEFT BREAST

Findings

In the subareolar area is a small, dense, spiculated mass (E7,M7). Directly posterior, there are two large oval masses (B5 and K4,L5), which are superimposed in the oblique view.

Discussion

Breast sonography showed that the oval masses were fluid-filled. Needle aspiration yielded clear fluid. In a woman of 69 years, fluid-filled masses are unusual, but in this case the cysts were attributed to the previous surgery. The spiculated density in the subareolar area *(Figure 13.3)* was thought to most likely represent a surgical scar. However, because of the history of carcinoma in situ at this same location, the possibility of recurrent tumor could not be ruled out. Excisional biopsy of the spiculated density revealed typical findings of a postoperative scar *(Figure 13.4)*.

Mammographic abnormalities after surgery include skin thickening and deformity, architectural distortion, and parenchymal scars, consisting of poorly defined masses often with spiculated margins.[134] While surgical scars may closely resemble carcinoma in mammograms, there are some important clues to the correct diagnosis. Scars tend to vary in shape in different mammographic projections, whereas tumors tend to maintain the same configuration. For example, in this case the spiculated density was round in the mediolateral projection but was elongate on the cephalocaudal. A baseline mammogram performed a few months after a biopsy could prove helpful, since a scar usually decreases in size in subsequent mammograms whereas a carcinoma would become larger. Scars are usually nonpalpable or can be felt only as a vague thickening despite relatively large size on the mammogram.

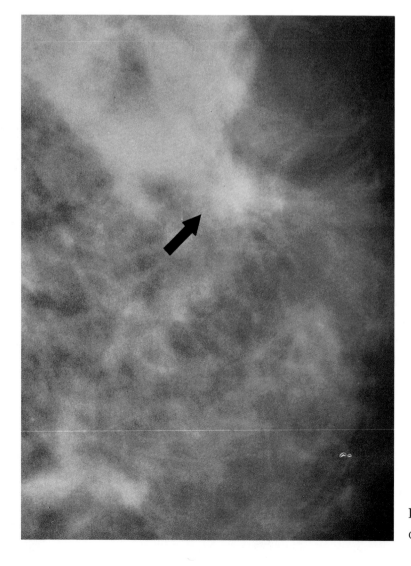

Figure 13.3

Close-up of spiculated mass.

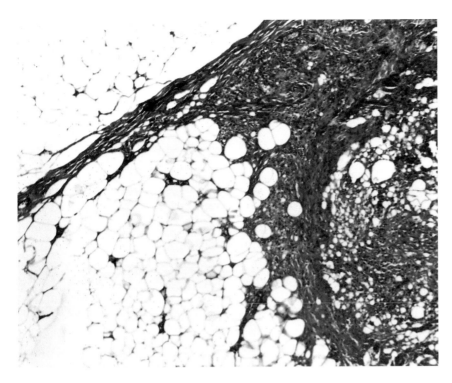

Figure 13.4

Low-power histologic section. Fibrosis extends into the surrounding fat,
resulting in the spiculations in the mammograms.

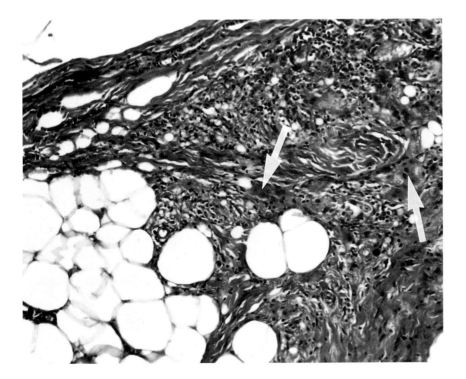

Figure 13.5

High-power histologic section. The center of the lesion shows chronic
inflammation with multinucleate giant cells (arrows). **Diagnosis**: Postbiopsy
scar.

Case 14

This 57-year-old woman presented with a right axillary mass and a left upper–outer quadrant mass.

Films: Right *(Figure 14.1)* and left *(Figure 14.2)* mediolateral oblique mammograms.

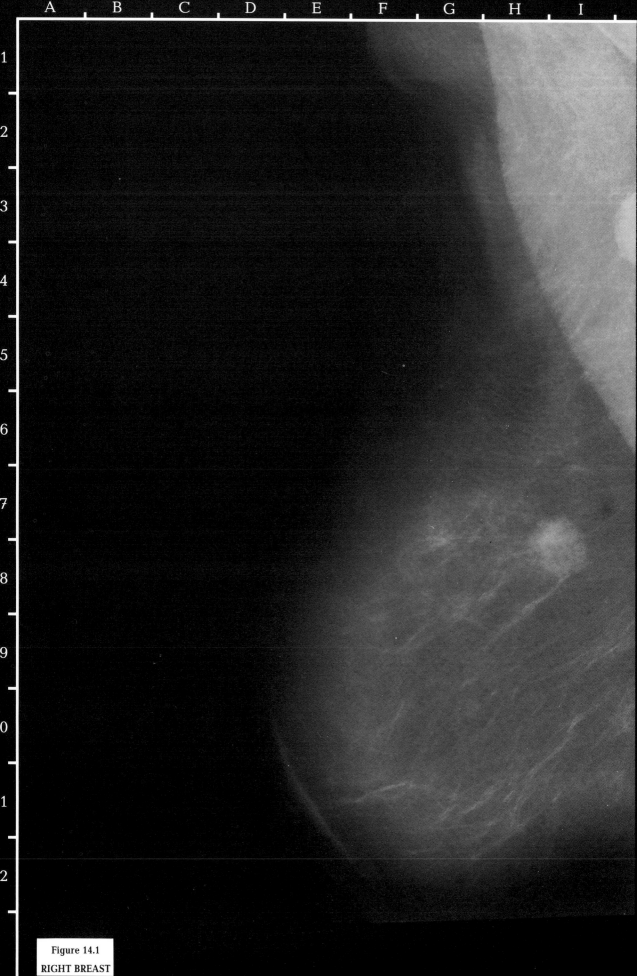

Figure 14.1
RIGHT BREAST

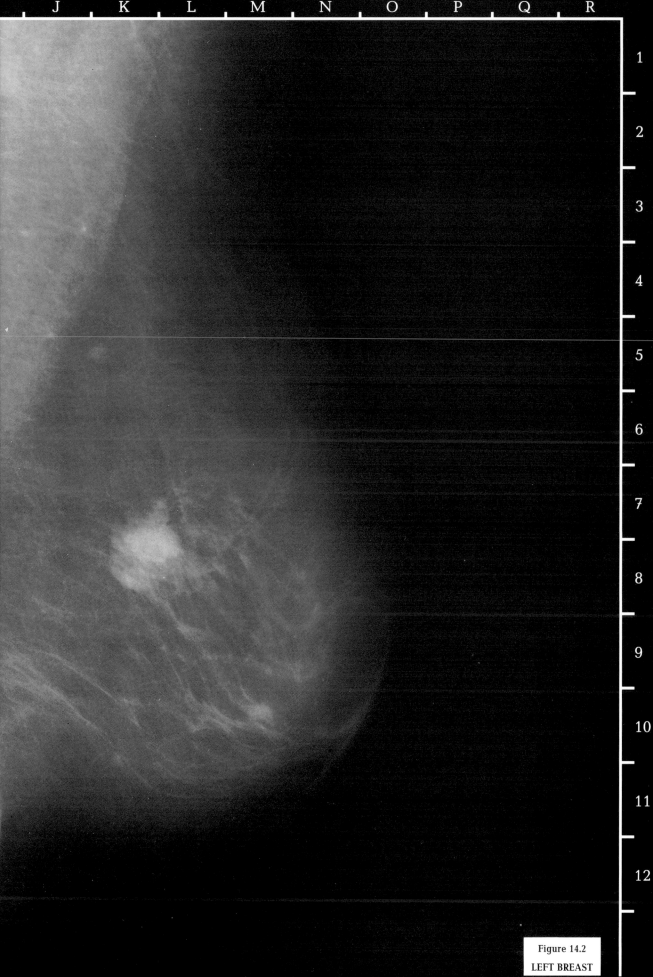

Figure 14.2
LEFT BREAST

Findings

A 2 cm dense mass (I3) is seen in the right axilla, and a poorly circumscribed 1.5 cm low-density mass is seen in the upper hemisphere of the right breast (I8). The left breast contains a dense, irregular, 2 cm mass (K8).

Discussion

Cephalocaudal views *(Figures 14.3 and 14.4)* show the bilateral breast masses. The right breast mass was not palpable, even though the examiner knew its location from the mammograms. Both right and left breast masses were suspicious for

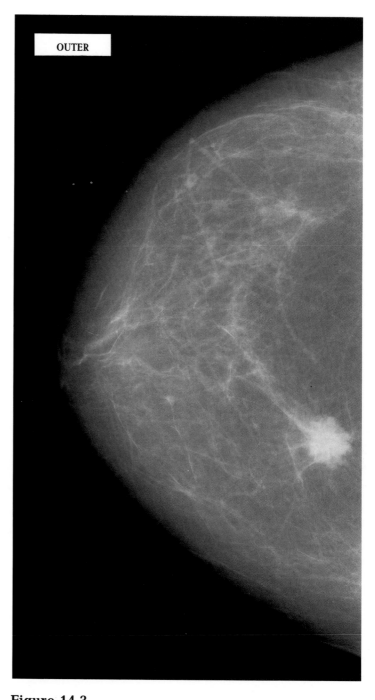

Figure 14.3

Cephalocaudal mammogram of right breast. Nonpalpable 1.5 cm mass shows spiculated margin.

malignancy. The prominent ducts anterior to the left breast mass may contain tumor or increased fibrous tissue.

Histologic examination of the biopsy specimens revealed bilateral infiltrating ductal carcinoma. The lymph node in the right axilla contained malignant cells. The patient had bilateral local excision of the masses, radiotherapy and chemotherapy.

The exact incidence of bilateral breast carcinoma is difficult to determine because it is not always possible to define whether a second

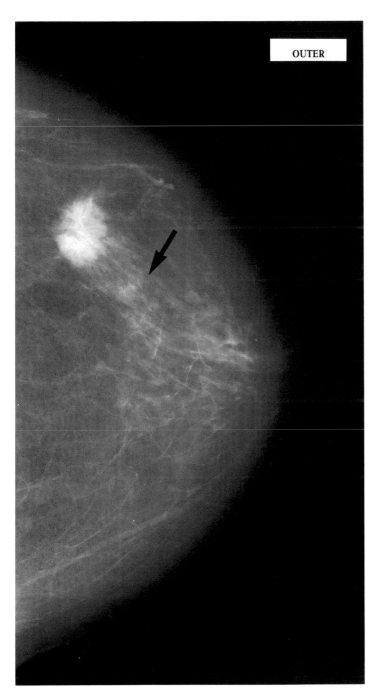

Figure 14.4

Cephalocaudal mammogram of left breast. The 2 cm mass is dense and spiculated. Ducts (arrow) anterior to mass are enlarged.

carcinoma was a primary tumor or metastatic from the contralateral breast. The incidence also depends on whether the cancers are detected by physical examination or mammography. The frequency of detection of synchronous bilateral tumors is enhanced by the use of mammography.[24] In one series of 172 biopsy-proved carcinomas, 87 (50.6 percent) were non-palpable at the time of mammography and 3 (1.7 percent) were mammographically bilateral.[12]

Case 15

The same patient as in Case 14 returned 7 months later with a palpable mass in the left breast.

Films: Right *(Figure 15.1)* and left *(Figure 15.2)* mediolateral mammograms.

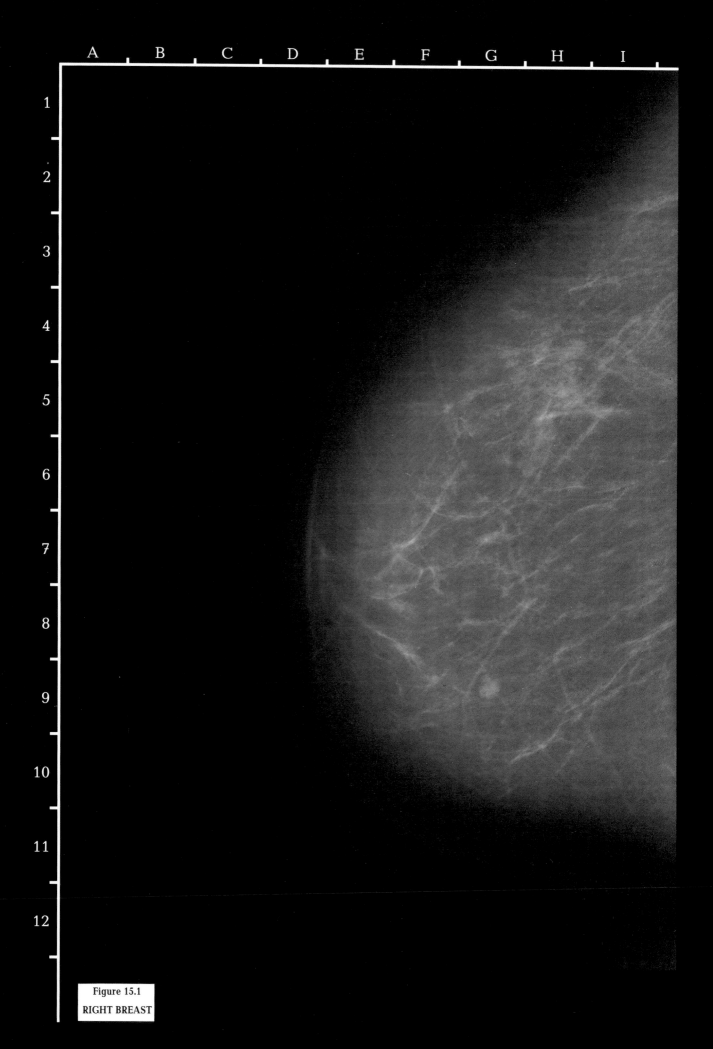

Figure 15.1
RIGHT BREAST

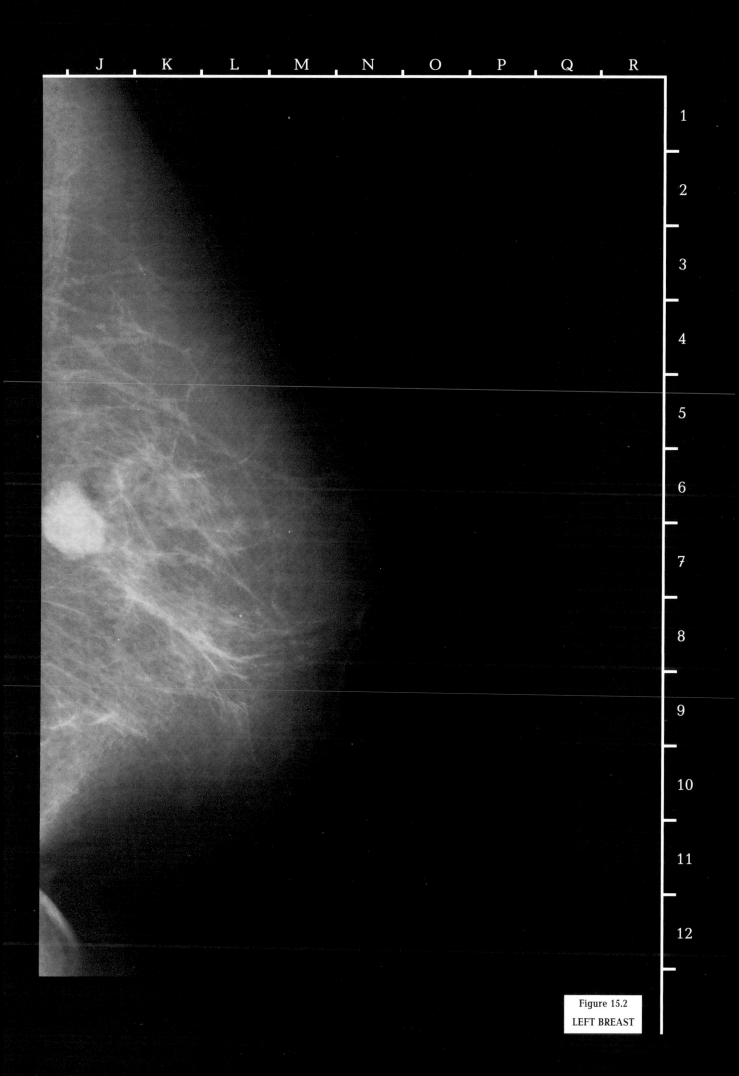

J   K   L   M   N   O   P   Q   R

1
2
3
4
5
6
7
8
9
10
11
12

Figure 15.2
LEFT BREAST

Findings

A 5 mm benign-appearing density (G9) in the right breast was present in the previous examination and has not changed. A 2 cm dense mass (J6) in the left breast has margins that are smooth posteriorly but somewhat irregular anteriorly.

Discussion

The cephalocaudal view confirms the ill-defined anterior margins of the left breast lesion *(Figure 15.3)*. Physical examination revealed a firm mass in the left upper–outer quadrant, at the site of the mammographic lesion. A mammogram performed

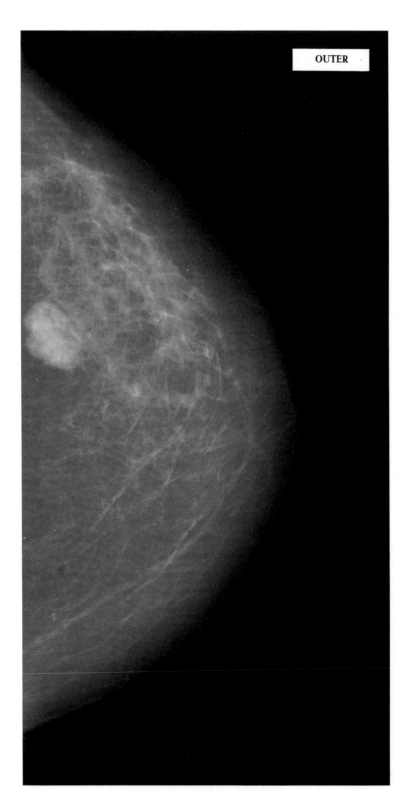

OUTER

Figure 15.3

Cephalocaudal mammogram of left breast shows a mass.

6 months earlier revealed no mass *(Figure 15.4)*. Recurrent breast cancer was suspected, and a biopsy was recommended. Histologic sections showed infiltrating ductal carcinoma.·

The risk of local recurrence after local excision and radiotherapy is estimated to be 2 percent per year for every year beyond therapy.[57] Three-quarters of recurrent cancers following radiotherapy will occur within the original tumor bed or within the area of previous segmental mastectomy.[111] In a study of 45 cases of biopsy-proven recurrence, 35 percent were detected by mammography alone, 39 percent by physical examination alone and 26 percent by both modalities.[141]

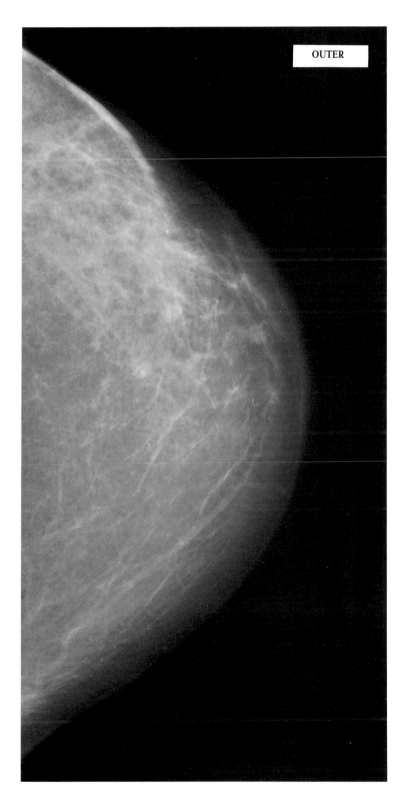

OUTER

Figure 15.4

Cephalocaudal mammogram of left breast performed 6 months prior to Figure 15.3. There is thickening and deformity of the skin at the site of the surgical excision. The mass was not present.

Benign mammographic changes that may occur after local excision and radiotherapy include thickening and retraction of the skin, increased parenchymal density, coarse calcifications, a mass and architectural distortion.[19,86] Mammographic evidence of tumor recurrence includes masses, microcalcifications and architectural distortion.[141]

Case 16

This 71-year-old woman was referred for a screening mammogram.

Films: Right *(Figure 16.1)* and left *(Figure 16.2)* mediolateral mammograms, and right *(Figure 16.3)* and left *(Figure 16.4)* cephalocaudal mammograms.

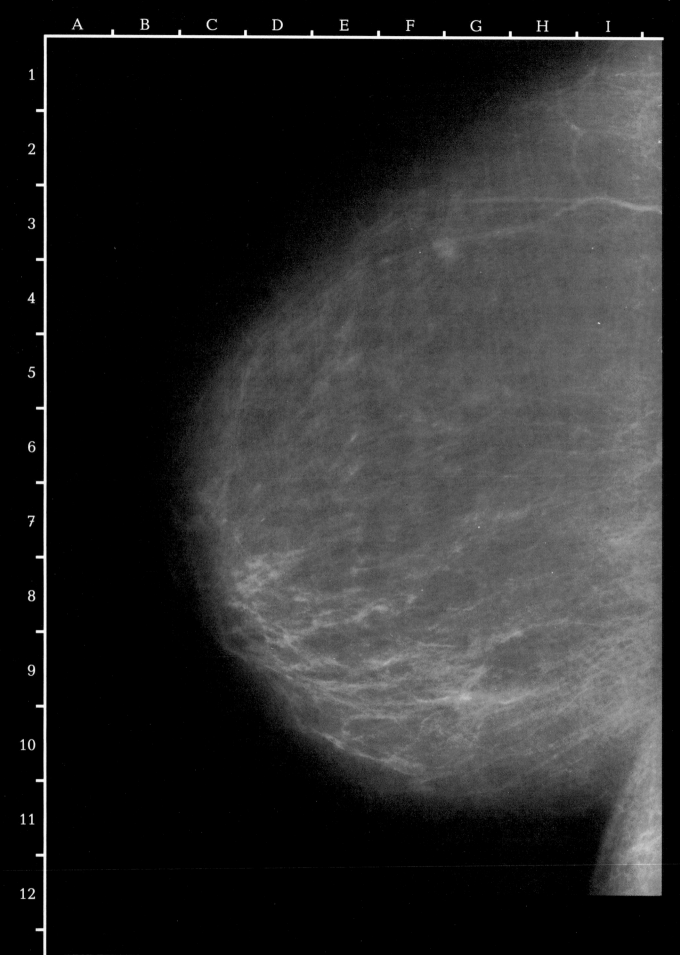

Figure 16.1
RIGHT BREAST

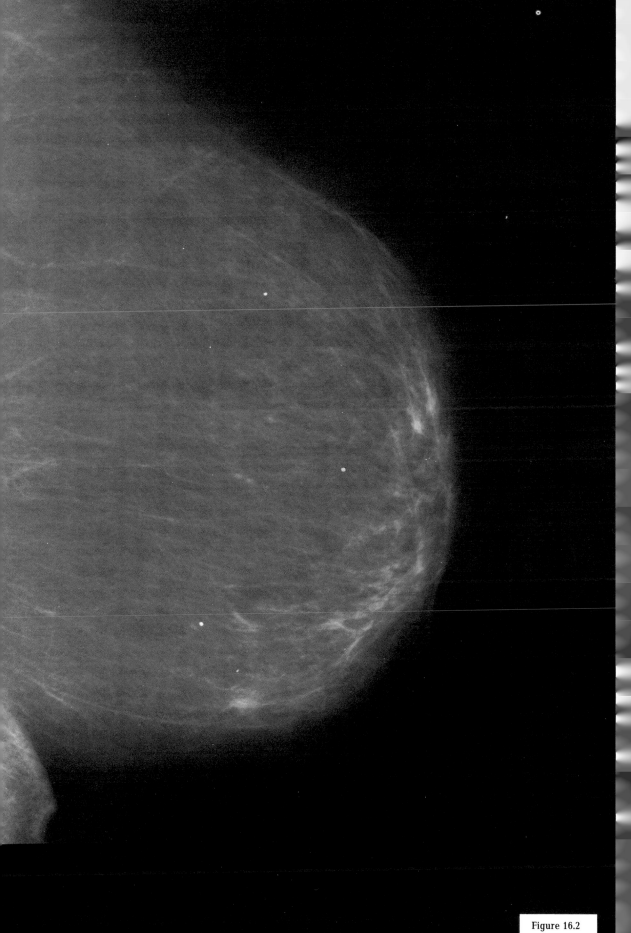

Figure 16.2
LEFT BREAST

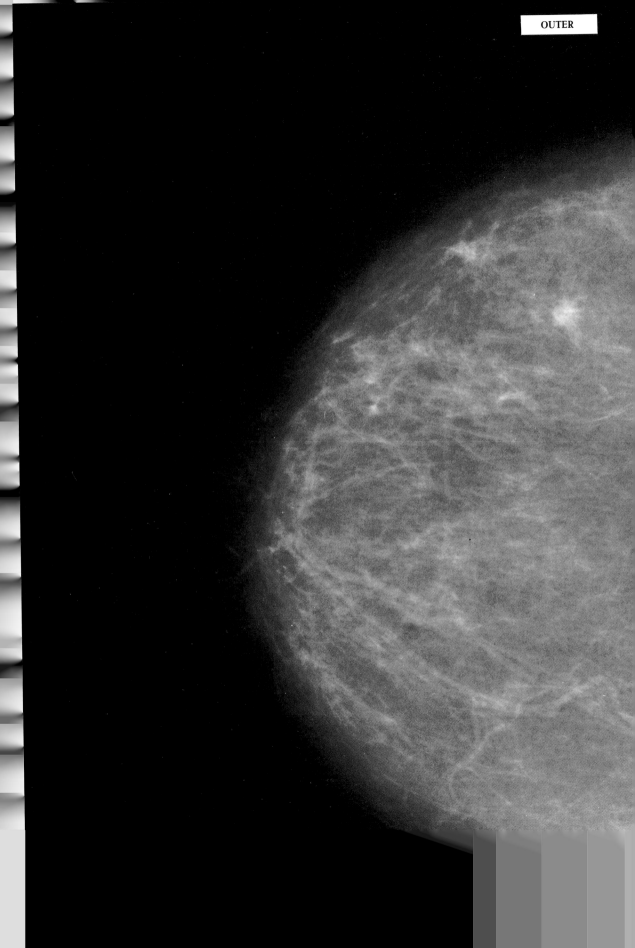

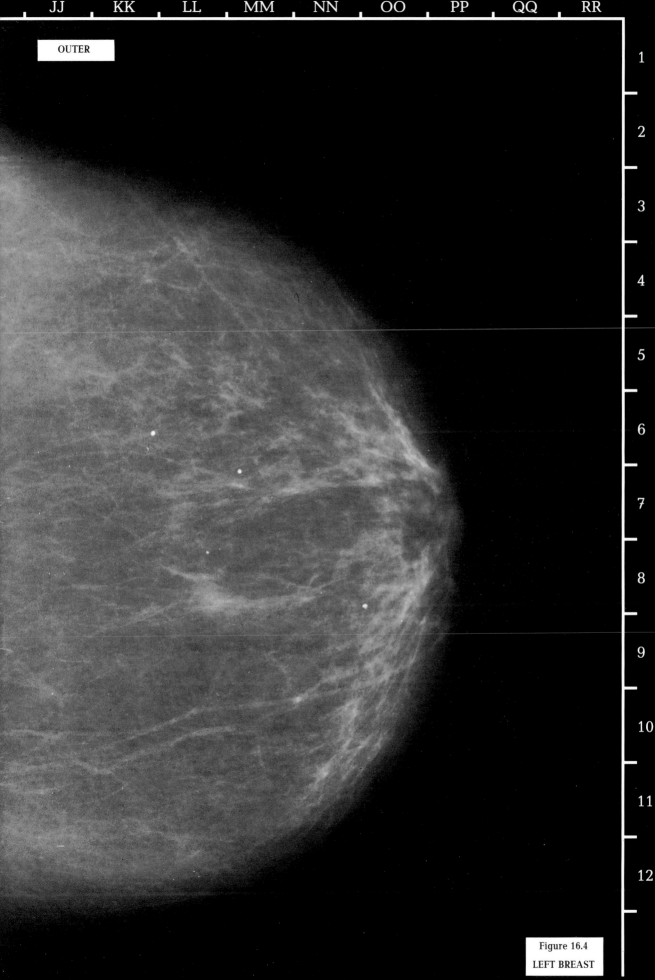

JJ   KK   LL   MM   NN   OO   PP   QQ   RR

OUTER

1
2
3
4
5
6
7
8
9
10
11
12

Figure 16.4
LEFT BREAST

Findings

In the right mediolateral view *(Figure 16.1)*, there is an ill-defined 7 mm density (G3) in the upper hemisphere. The right cephalocaudal view *(Figure 16.3)* confirms the presence of the density (II5), and localizes it to the upper–outer quadrant.

In the left mediolateral view *(Figure 16.2)*, an ill-defined 5 mm density (M10) is seen in the lower hemisphere. In the left cephalocaudal view *(Figure 16.4)*, the density is difficult to identify but may lie posterior to the nipple (LL8).

Discussion

In order to improve the depiction of these small densities, 'spot' or 'coned' compression views of both breasts *(Figures 16.5 and 16.6)* were performed. The density in the left breast cannot be confirmed in the spot views. The density in the right breast has suspicious peripheral spiculations and biopsy revealed infiltrating ductal carcinoma *(Figure 16.7)*.

This case illustrates the value of spot compression in the confirmation or exclusion of the presence of equivocal abnormalities. In one series of 46 possible masses, spot compression showed that 39 were fictitious, supported the biopsy of 2 carcinomas, and confirmed the benign features of 2 masses.[18] By displacement of the overlying breast tissue, diminution of the area of X-ray exposure with appropriate coning, and decrease of the breast thickness in the area of interest, the small spot-compression device further diminishes scattered radiation, and thereby allows for better depiction of masses and calcifications.

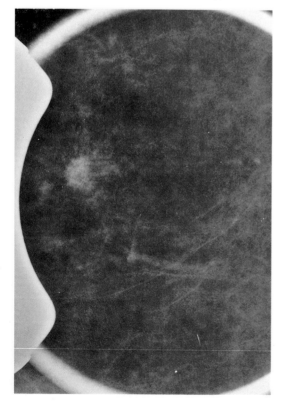

Figure 16.5

Spot compression, cephalocaudal projection, shows irregular margin of 7 mm right breast mass.

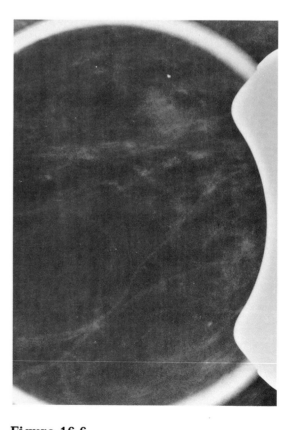

Figure 16.6

Spot compression, cephalocaudal projection, excludes a left breast mass.

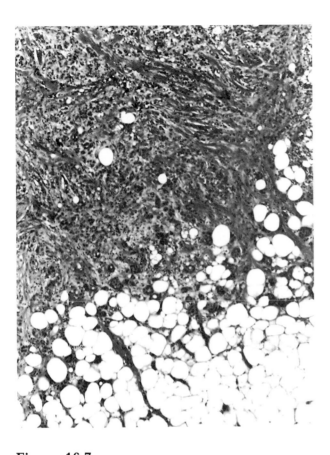

Figure 16.7

Low-power histologic section of right breast mass.
Malignant ductal epithelial cells invade the
surrounding fat and create an irregular boundary.
Marked desmoplasia is present. **Diagnosis**: Infiltrating
ductal carcinoma.

Case 17

A 63-year-old woman was referred for a screening mammogram.

Films: Cephalocaudal views of the right *(Figure 17.1)* and left *(Figure 17.2)* breasts.

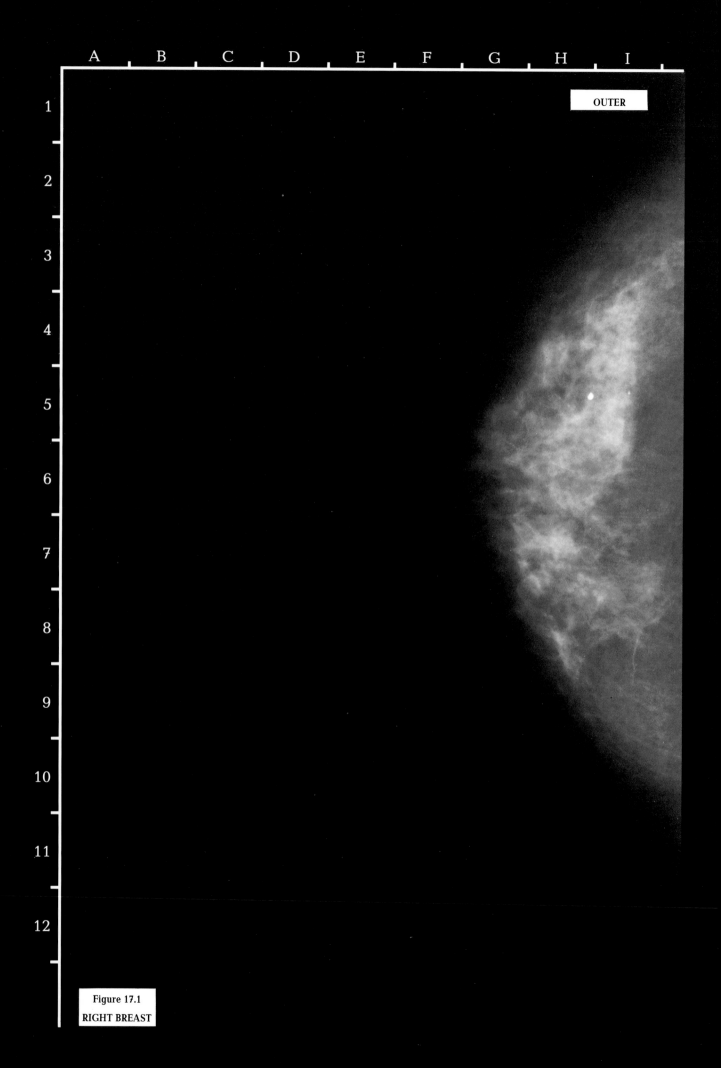

OUTER

Figure 17.1
RIGHT BREAST

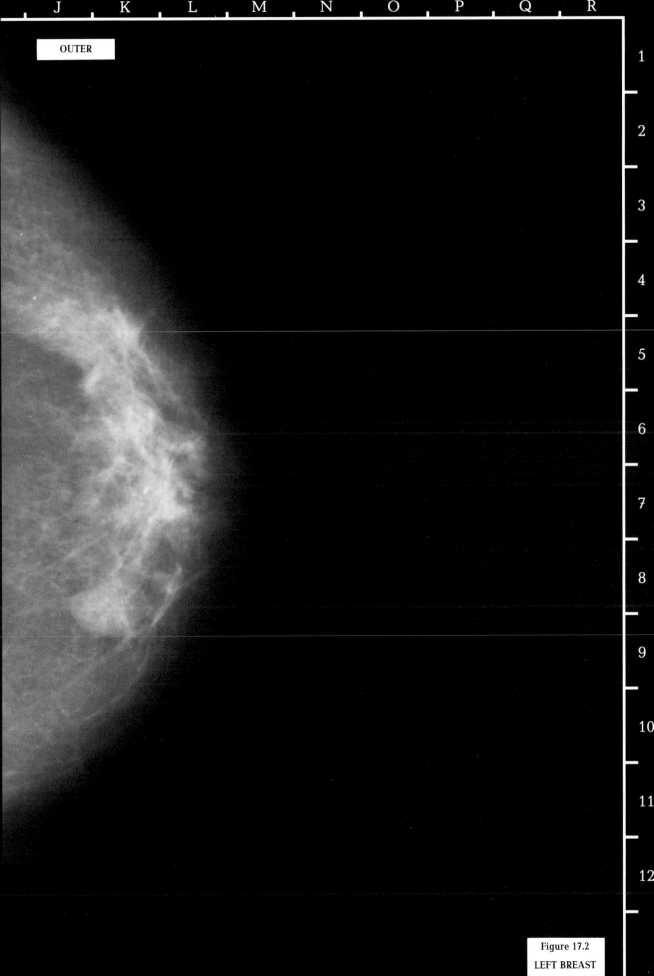

OUTER

Figure 17.2
LEFT BREAST

Findings

Two benign-appearing calcifications are present on the right. An intermediate-density mass (J9) is located in the inner hemisphere of the left breast.

Discussion

The mediolateral view *(Figure 17.3)* confirms the presence of the left breast lesion. A spot-compression view *(Figure 17.4)* shows a discrete, dense mass with ill-defined borders. A biopsy was performed *(Figure 17.5)*. The pathologic diagnosis was localized fibrosis *(Figure. 17.6 and 17.7)*.

Isolated fibrosis of the breast is a distinct clinicopathologic entity characterized by stromal fibrosis and obliteration of the lobular and ductal structures. It tends to occur in women of 35–49 years of age, and is usually unilateral, most often in the upper–outer quadrant.[54] It usually presents as a palpable mass, but may also be detected as a dense nonpalpable mass in a screening mammogram.[59] When palpable, fibrosis is characterized as a hard, painless tumor similar to malignancy. The incidence of isolated fibrosis is reported to be 7.9 percent of surgically resected breast specimens.[117] Fibrosis may also accompany fibrocystic changes.

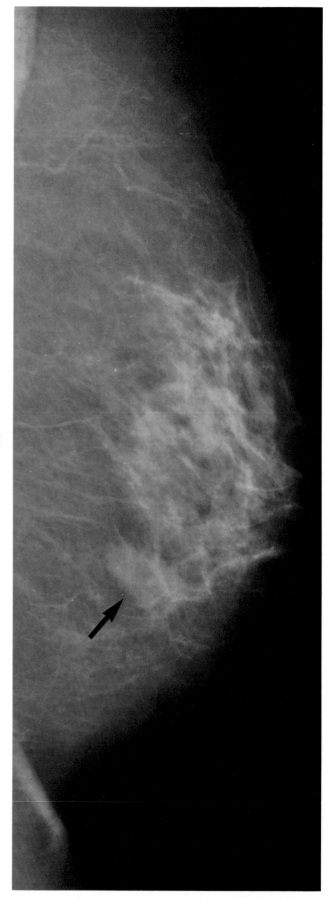

Figure 17.3

Mediolateral view of left breast shows the density (arrow) in the lower hemisphere.

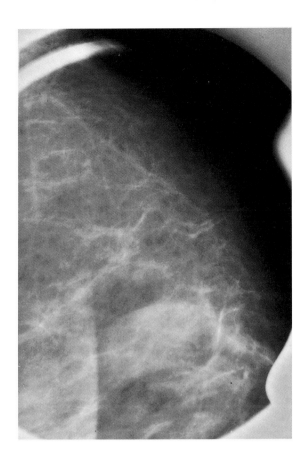

Figure 17.4

Spot compression. The lesion is dense and has ill-defined margins.

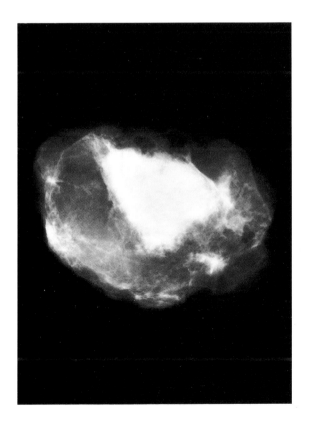

Figure 17.5

Specimen radiograph.

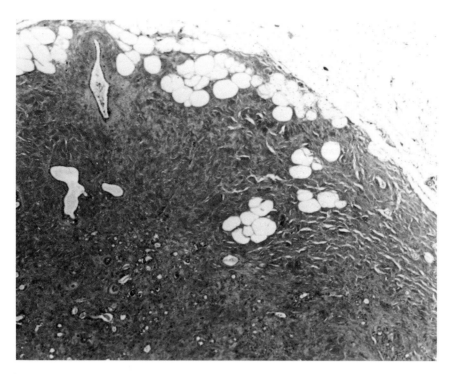

Figure 17.6

Low-power histologic section. The lesion is well demarcated from surrounding adipose tissue and is characterized by stromal fibrous tissue overgrowth. **Diagnosis**: Fibrosis.

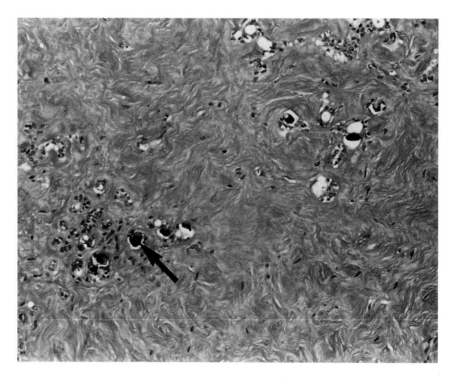

Figure 17.7

High-power histologic section. Foci of calcification (arrow) noted within the benign atrophic lobules were not depicted in the mammograms.

Case 18

A 57-year-old asymptomatic woman was referred for 'a suspicious abnormality in the left breast' detected on screening mammograms.

Film: Left mediolateral oblique view *(Figure 18.1).*

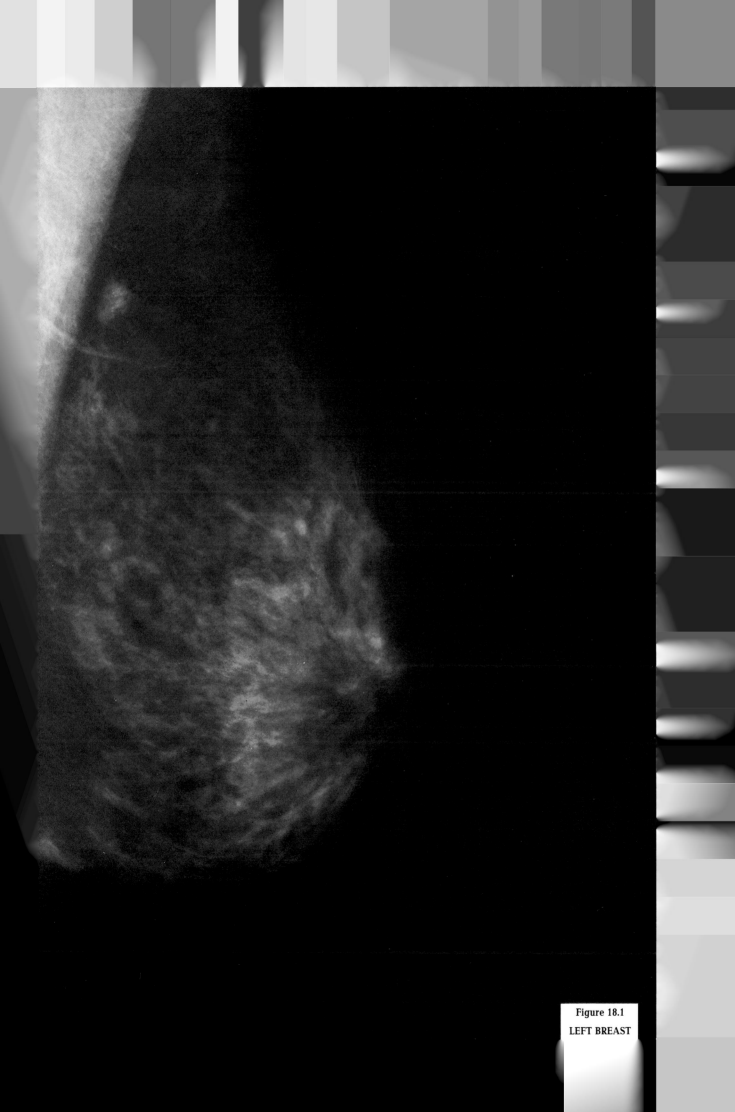

Figure 18.1
LEFT BREAST

Findings

There is a lobulated mass (J3) in the upper hemisphere of the breast, just anterior to the pectoral muscle. Numerous microcalcifications are present within the mass.

Discussion

Because carcinoma was suspected, a biopsy was performed *(Figure 18.2)*. The pathology revealed a degenerating fibroadenoma *(Figure 18.3)*.

After menopause, fibroadenomas undergo atrophy and frequently calcify. The calcifications typically are coarse, often shaped like popcorn, and few in number. Less commonly, as in this case, they may mimic the microcalcifications of carcinoma.

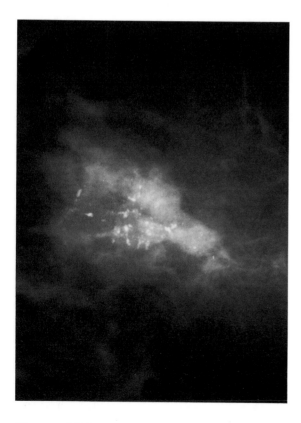

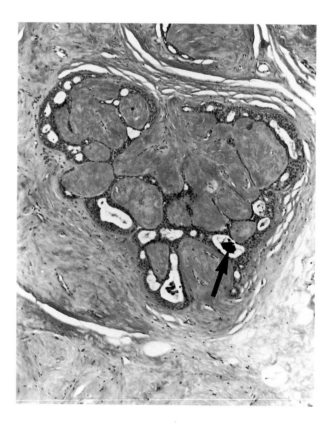

Figure 18.2

Specimen radiograph shows numerous calcifications within the mass. The calcifications are suspicious for malignancy: they are numerous, clustered, vary in size and shape, are linear and have a branching distribution.

Figure 18.3

Low-power histologic section from center of mass. Compressed branching ducts within a fibrous stroma are characteristic of fibroadenoma. Calcification (arrow) is demonstrated within the lumen of a duct within the fibroadenoma.

Case 19

This 61-year-old woman had had a left tylectomy (lumpectomy) and radiotherapy for carcinoma 2 years prior to these mammograms. She complained of a right upper–outer quadrant mass.

Films: Right *(Figure 19.1)* and left *(Figure 19.2)* cephalocaudal mammograms.

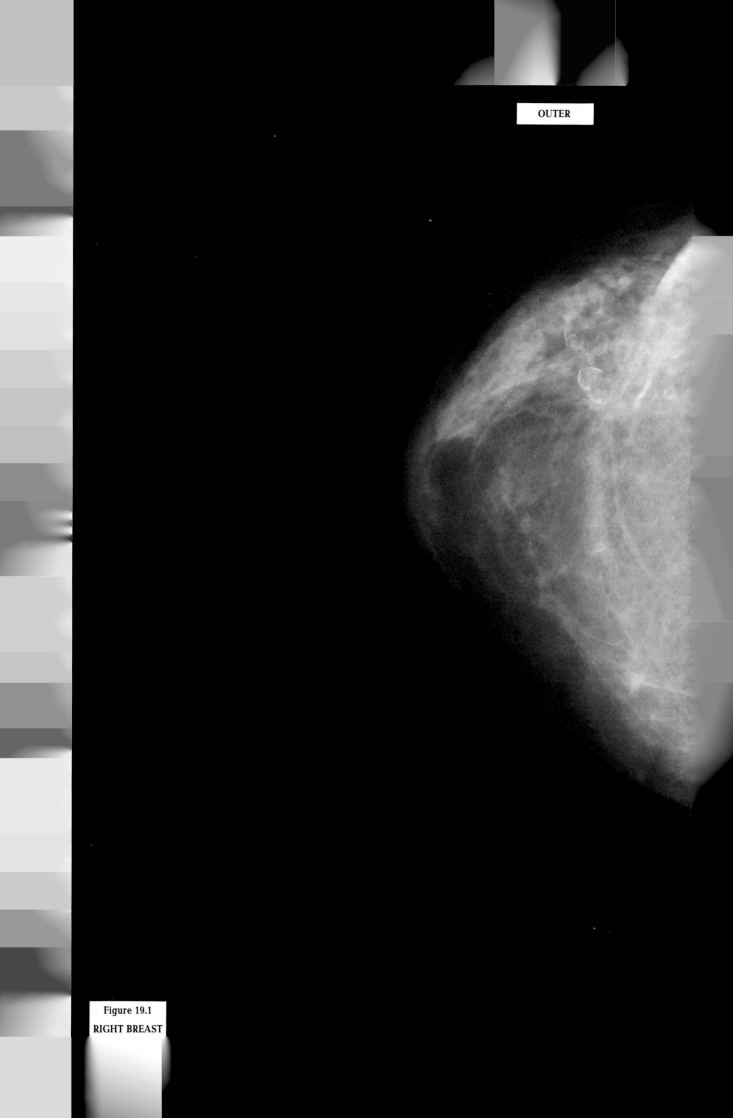

OUTER

Figure 19.1
RIGHT BREAST

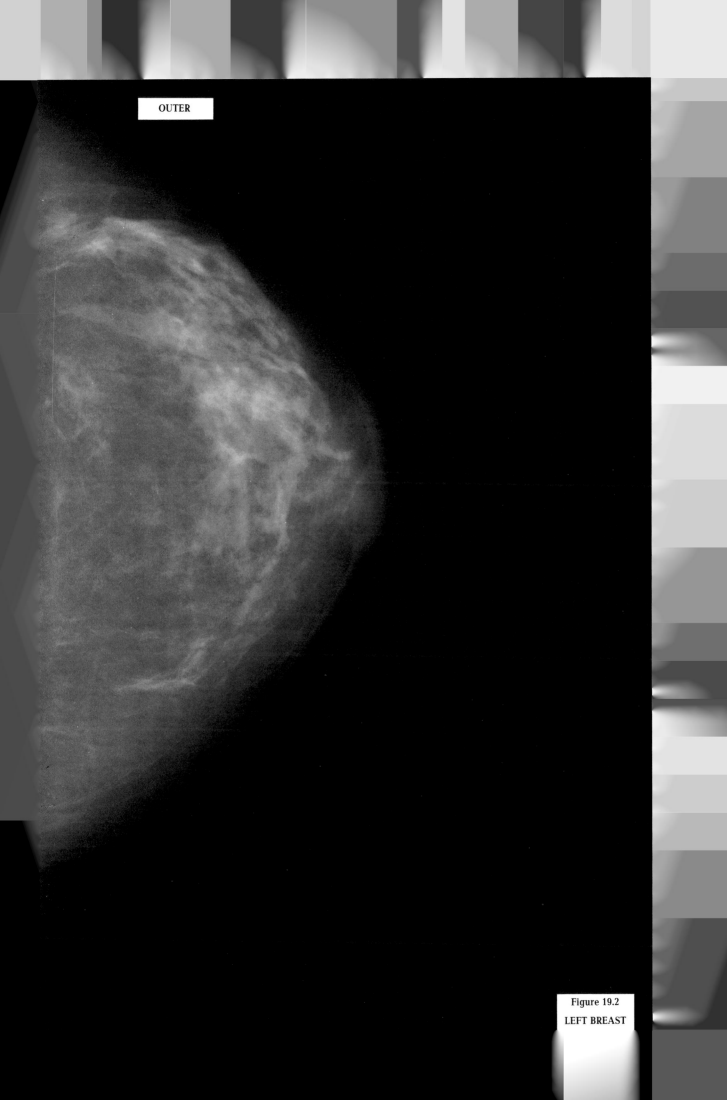

OUTER

Figure 19.2

LEFT BREAST

Findings

There is generalized skin thickening and localized deformity of the skin at the biopsy site (I3). In addition, numerous fat-density cyst-like lesions are surrounded by rings of calcification (H4).

Discussion

The mammograms *(Figure 19.3)* show one of the typical mammographic features of fat necrosis: calcified lipid-filled (oil) cysts. The spectrum of mammographic features includes a spiculated

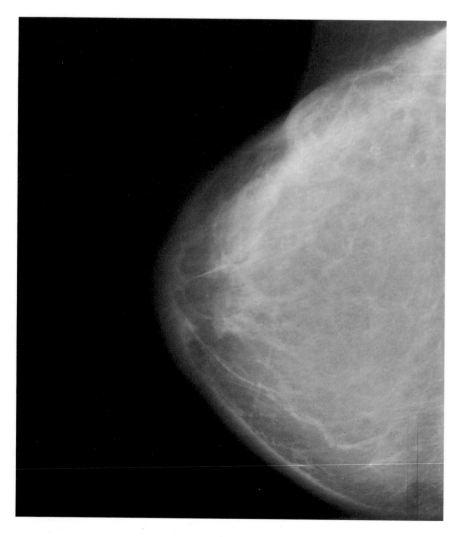

Figure 19.3

Close-up of mediolateral oblique view of the right breast. Ring-like calcifications are present under the thickened, retracted skin at the biopsy site.

mass, skin thickening and retraction, oil cysts, and microcalcifications which may mimic those of malignancy but which usually are benign in appearance as in this case.[2,14,15,102] Despite the characteristic mammographic features, a biopsy of the palpable mass was performed and the diagnosis of fat necrosis was confirmed histologically *(Figure 19.4).*

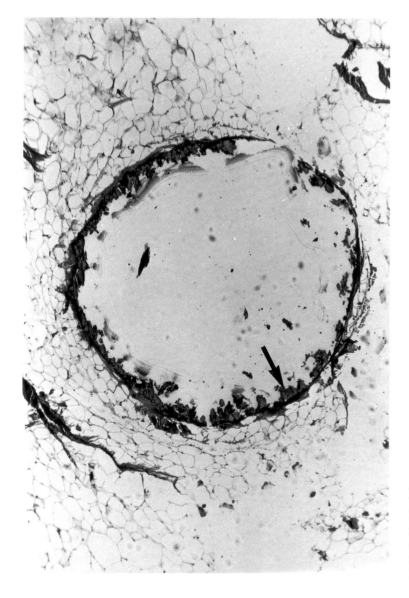

Figure 19.4

Low-power histologic section. Within the necrotic fat tissue is a spherical calcification (arrow) seen along the inner margin of an intact fibrous ring.
Diagnosis: Fat necrosis.

Case 20

A 44-year-old woman who had undergone a heart transplant 5 years earlier was referred for a palpable mass in the six o'clock position of the left breast. A mass was not palpable at the time of mammography.

Films: Right *(Figure 20.1)* and left *(Figure 20.2)* mediolateral oblique mammograms.

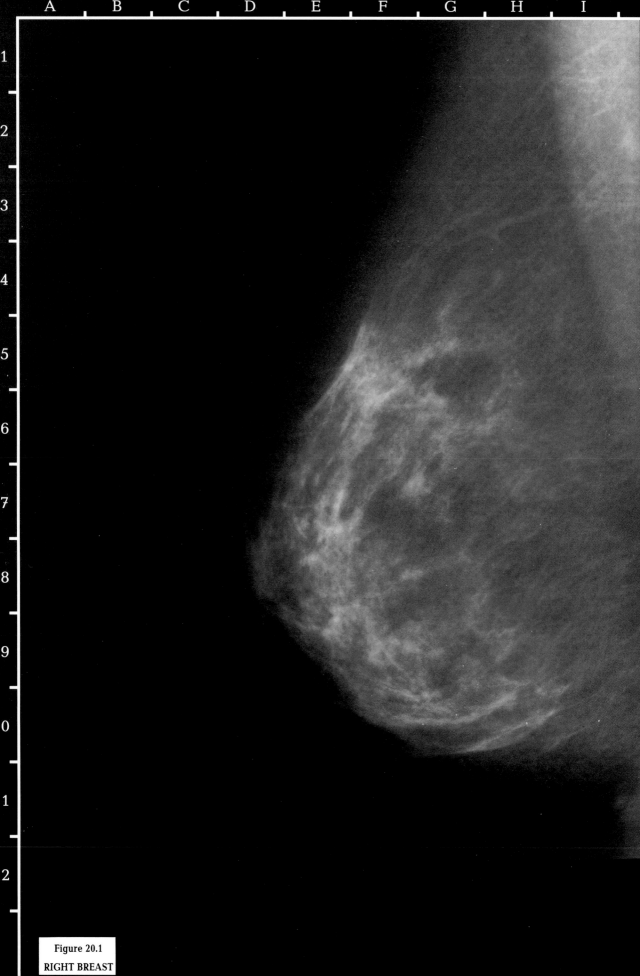

Figure 20.1
RIGHT BREAST

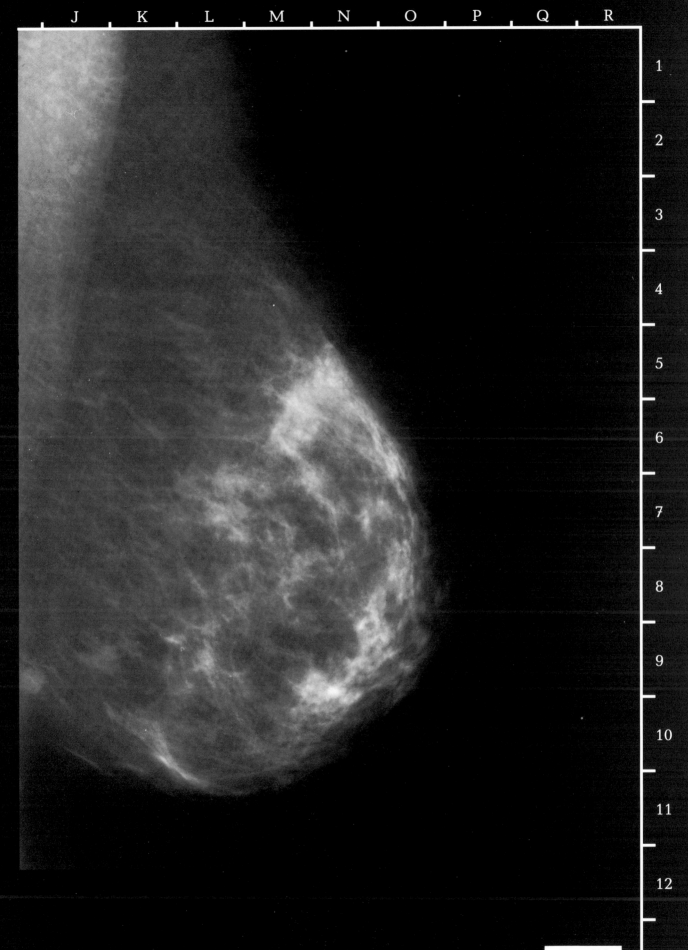

Figure 20.2
LEFT BREAST

Findings

There is a 7 mm well-defined nodule (J9) of intermediate density in the inferior hemisphere of the left breast, near the chest wall. The right breast shows no abnormality.

Discussion

The well-circumscribed margin was confirmed on the cephalocaudal view *(Figure 20.3)*. The mammographic impression was of a benign mass, most likely a cyst or fibroadenoma. Because sonography failed to show a cyst, a biopsy was performed *(Figure 20.4)*. Histology revealed poorly differentiated carcinoma with progesterone-receptor positivity, identifying this as a primary breast tumor *(Figure 20.5)*. Despite the small size and relatively smooth margins of the tumor, the patient died only a few months later of widely disseminated breast carcinoma.

A well-circumscribed solid mass should be considered for biopsy if it is palpable, solitary, growing, not present on a previous mammogram, and does not contain the typical coarse calcifications of a fibroadenoma.

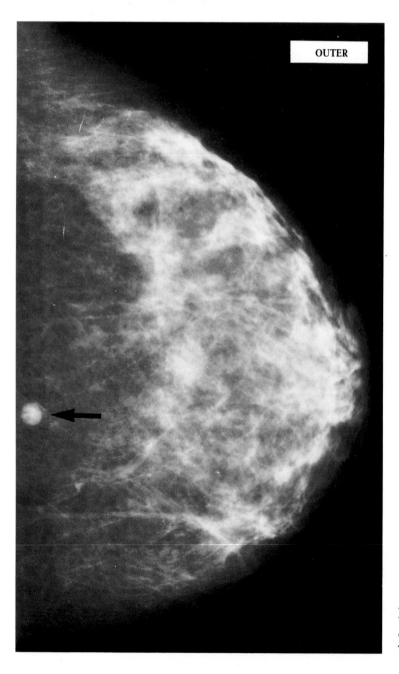

OUTER

Figure 20.3

Cephalocaudal mammogram of left breast. The nodule (arrow) has smooth margins.

This patient was on immunosuppressive therapy for her heart transplant. While there is an increased incidence of skin cancer, non-Hodgkin's lymphoma, Kaposi's sarcoma and primary liver cancer in patients who have undergone organ transplantation and cyclosporine therapy, there is no increased incidence of common tumors such as cancers of the lung, colon, prostate and breast.[113]

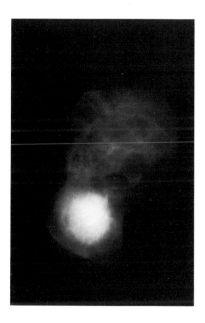

Figure 20.4

Specimen radiograph.

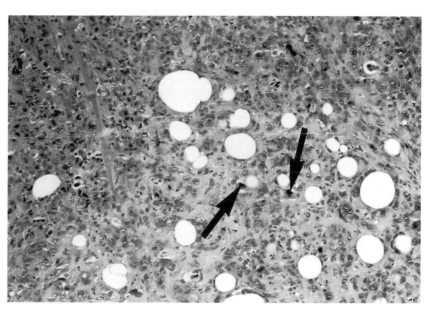

Figure 20.5

High-power histologic section. Nests and cords of neoplastic cells infiltrate a fibrous stroma. Numerous mitotic figures (arrows) are present.

Case 21

This 51-year-old woman complained of pain in the right breast.

Films: Right *(Figure 21.1)* and left *(Figure 21.2)* mediolateral oblique mammograms.

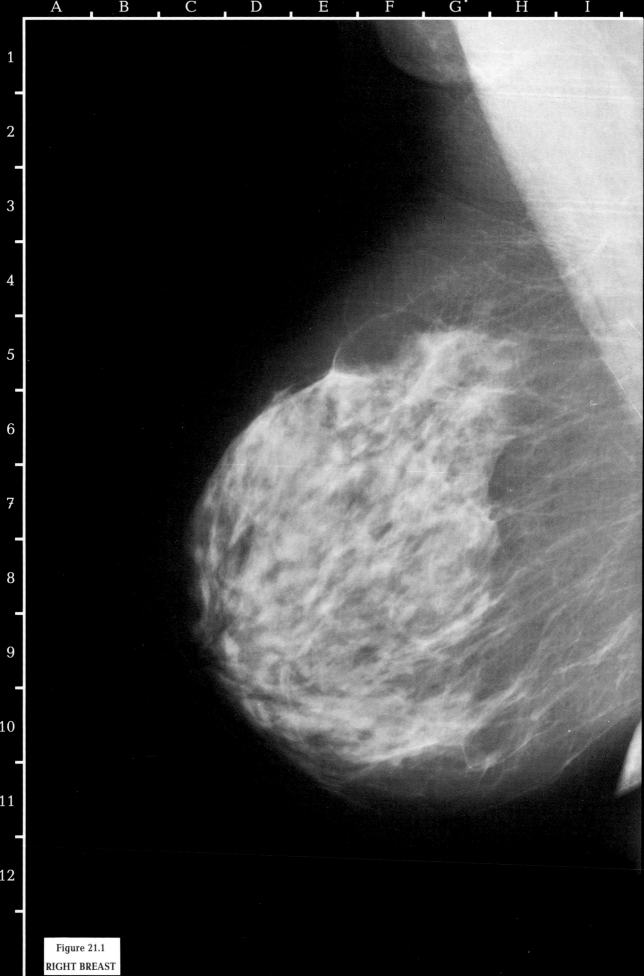

Figure 21.1
RIGHT BREAST

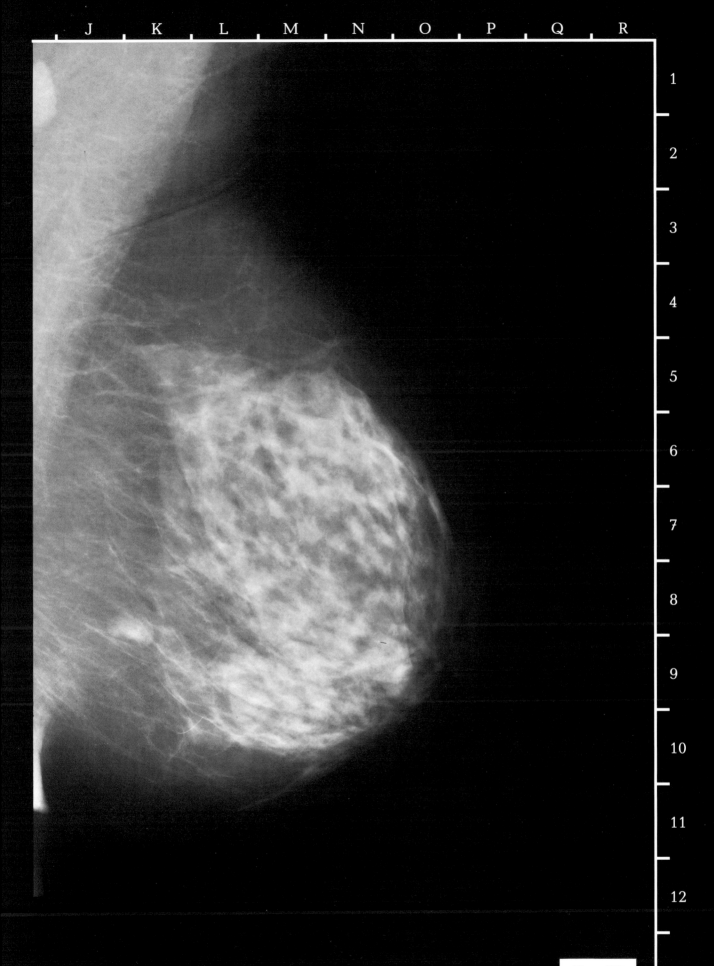

Figure 21.2

LEFT BREAST

Findings

There are prominent ducts and axillary lymph nodes bilaterally. An 8 mm by 13 mm mass (K8) is present in the left breast.

Discussion

In the cephalocaudal view of the left breast the mass is located in the inner hemisphere *(Figure 21.3)*. It could not be palpated. If the mass had been located within the dense parenchymal tissue, it most likely would have gone undetected in the mammograms. Because sonography showed that the mass was solid, a biopsy was recommended. Histologic examination revealed invasive lobular carcinoma.

A well-circumscribed mass is reported to be the least common mammographic presentation of infiltrating lobular carcinoma.[100] Its other mammographic manifestations are asymmetric density without a definable mass, high-density mass with spiculated borders, dense breast with no discernible tumor, and microcalcifications similar to those seen in infiltrating ductal carcinoma.

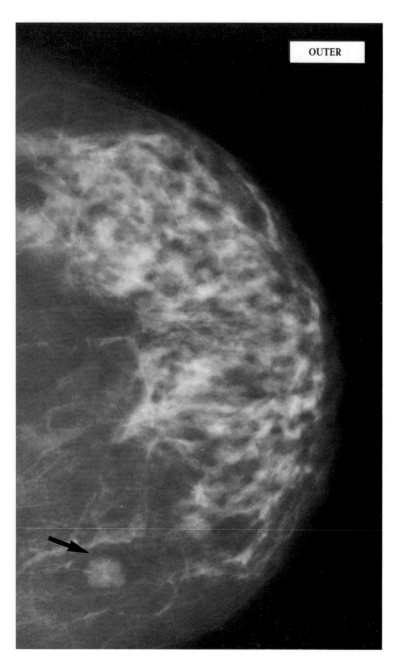

OUTER

Figure 21.3

Cephalocaudal mammogram of left breast. The mass (arrow) has relatively well-circumscribed margins. **Pathologic diagnosis**: Lobular carcinoma.

Case 22

A 56-year-old woman was referred for a screening mammogram.

Films: Right *(Figure 22.1)* and left *(Figure 22.2)* mediolateral mammograms.

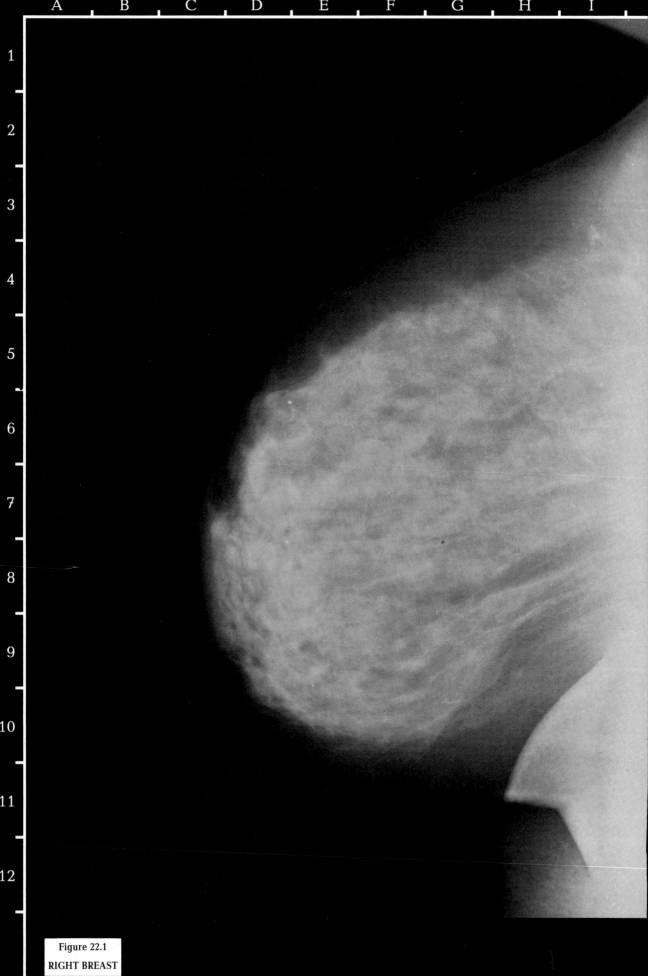

Figure 22.1
RIGHT BREAST

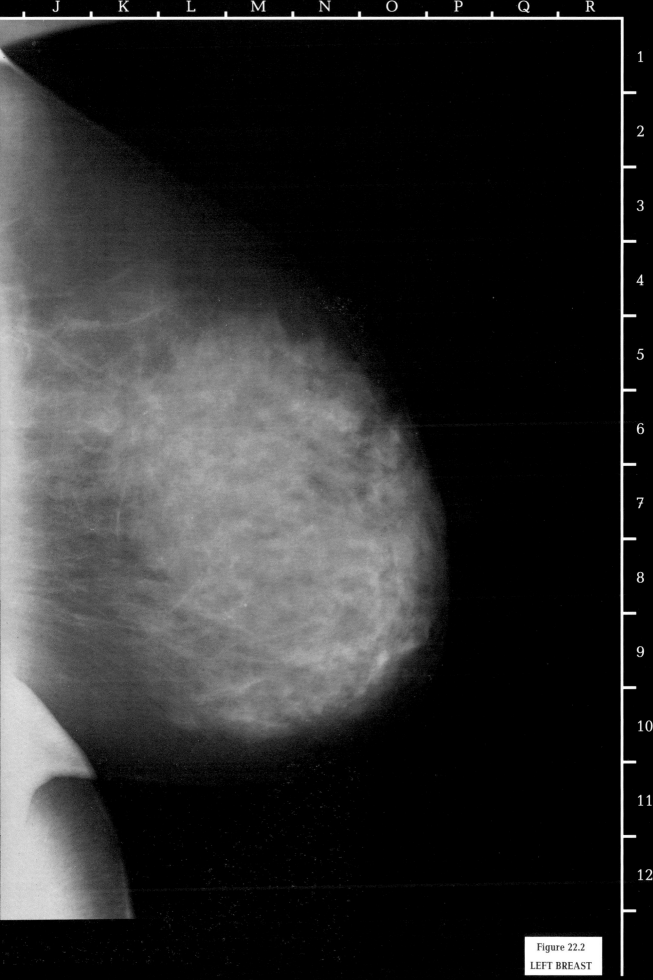

Figure 22.2
LEFT BREAST

Findings

The breasts are dense. An area of spiculated architectural distortion (K6) is present in the left upper hemisphere. The right breast is unremarkable.

Discussion

The cephalocaudal projections *(Figure 22.3 and 22.4)* verify the architectural irregularity, and localize it to the upper–outer quadrant of the left breast. There was no palpable abnormality and no

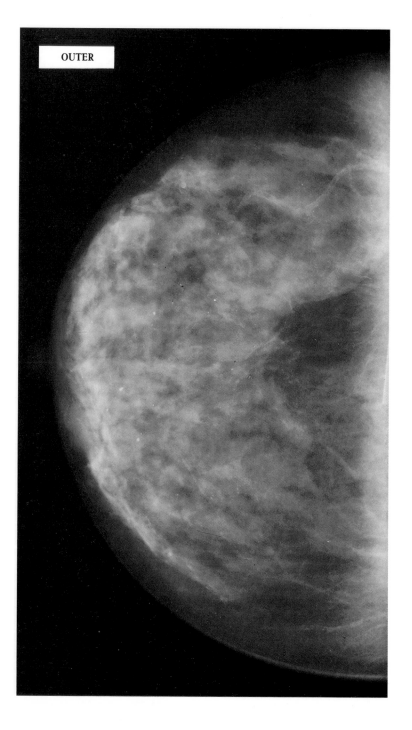

Figure 22.3

Cephalocaudal view of right breast shows no abnormality.

history of previous surgery. A biopsy was recommended, and revealed infiltrating ductal carcinoma *(Figure 22.5)*.

An architectural distortion may be the only sign of breast carcinoma.[105] The distortion should also be identified in a second projection to confirm its presence and to localize it. In this case, the distortion resulted from a desmoplastic response initiated by a carcinoma. Because similar parenchymal changes may follow surgery, it is important to be aware of the location of any surgical scars in interpretation of the mammograms.

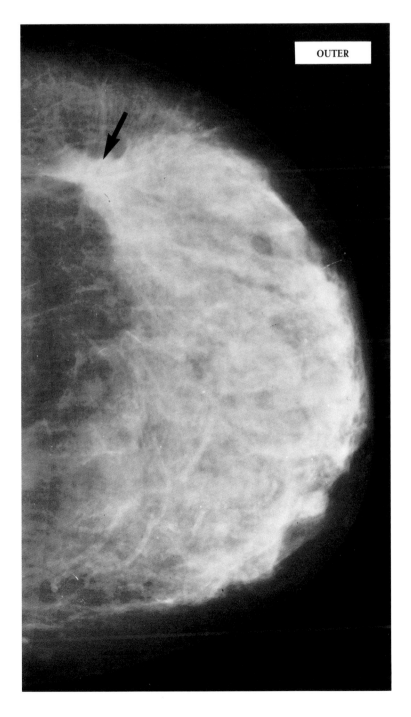

OUTER

Figure 22.4

Cephalocaudal view of left breast. The area of architectural distortion (arrow) previously seen is identified in the outer hemisphere.

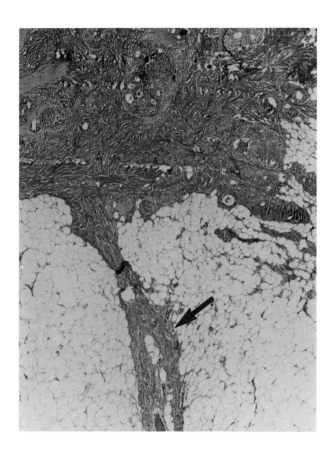

Figure 22.5

Low-power histologic section. Infiltrating ductal carcinoma with a radiating pattern of fibrosis produces a stellate configuration on the mammogram. A long spicule (arrow) of fibrous tissue is seen extending into the surrounding fat ('tail of comet' sign).

Case 23

This patient had a 1-month history of a lump in the left breast.

Films: Right *(Figure 23.1)* and left *(Figure 23.2)* cephalocaudal mammograms.

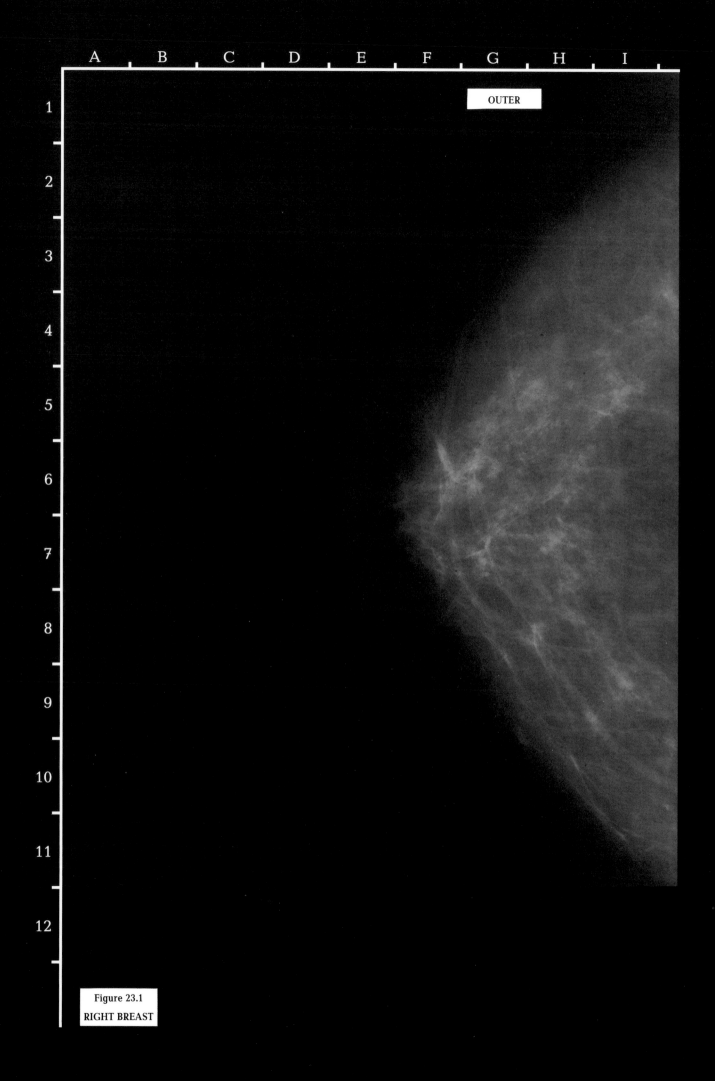

OUTER

Figure 23.1
RIGHT BREAST

OUTER

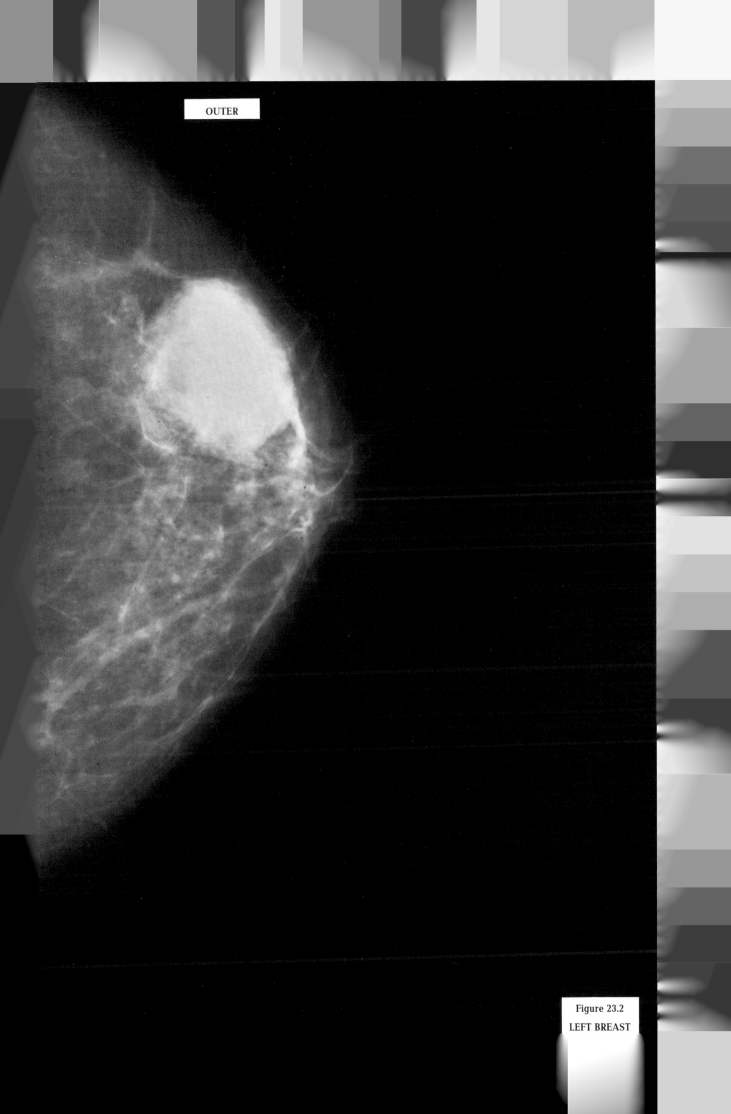

Figure 23.2
LEFT BREAST

Findings

There is a 4.5 × 3.5 cm mass in the left breast (L5).

Discussion

The margins of the mass are poorly defined posteriorly. Sonography showed that it was solid. Biopsy revealed cystosarcoma phyllodes *(Figure 23.3).*

Cystosarcoma phyllodes, like fibroadenoma, has both epithelial and stromal components. However, the stroma of cystosarcoma is more cellular and the cells vary more in size and shape. The average age of patients with cystosarcoma is 40.5 years.[54] In our experience, most cystosarcomas are nonmetastatic and have limited invasion into the surrounding breast parenchyma. They may grow to a very large size, causing distortion in the contour of the overlying skin, or even ulceration. Cystosarcomas have a high rate of recurrence if not completely excised. The reported incidence of malignant cystosarcoma varies among different series from 6 to 43 percent.[49,54] Metastatic potential is suggested by an increase in the mitotic rate (more than 3 per 10 high-power fields), invasion of adjacent breast tissue (infiltrating vs mere pushing) and size (over 4 cm).[107]

Mammographically, cystosarcomas are relatively well circumscribed, large and grow rapidly over serial examinations.[51] They are rarely calcified.

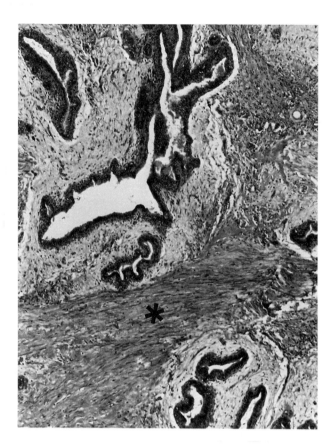

Figure 23.3

Low-power histologic section. Long, branching epithelium-lined clefts are surrounded by a cellular fibrous stroma (asterisk).

Diagnosis: Cystosarcoma phyllodes.

Case 24

A 46-year-old asymptomatic woman had a screening mammogram.

Films: Right *(Figure 24.1)* and left *(Figure 24.2)* mediolateral oblique mammograms.

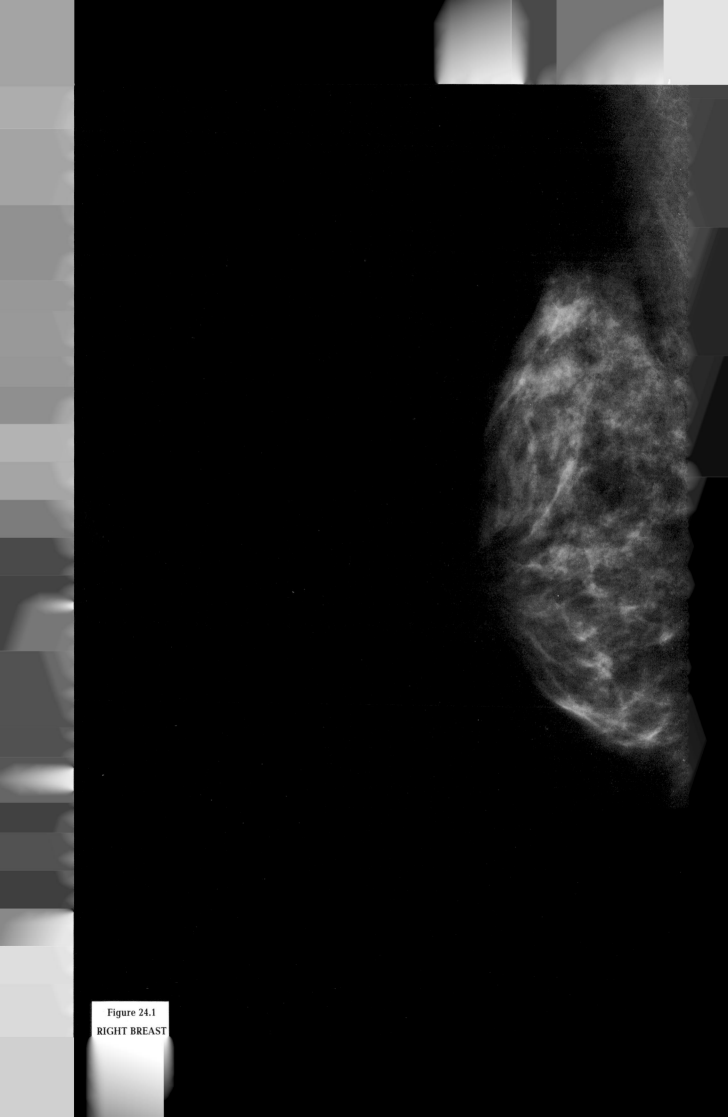

Figure 24.1
RIGHT BREAST

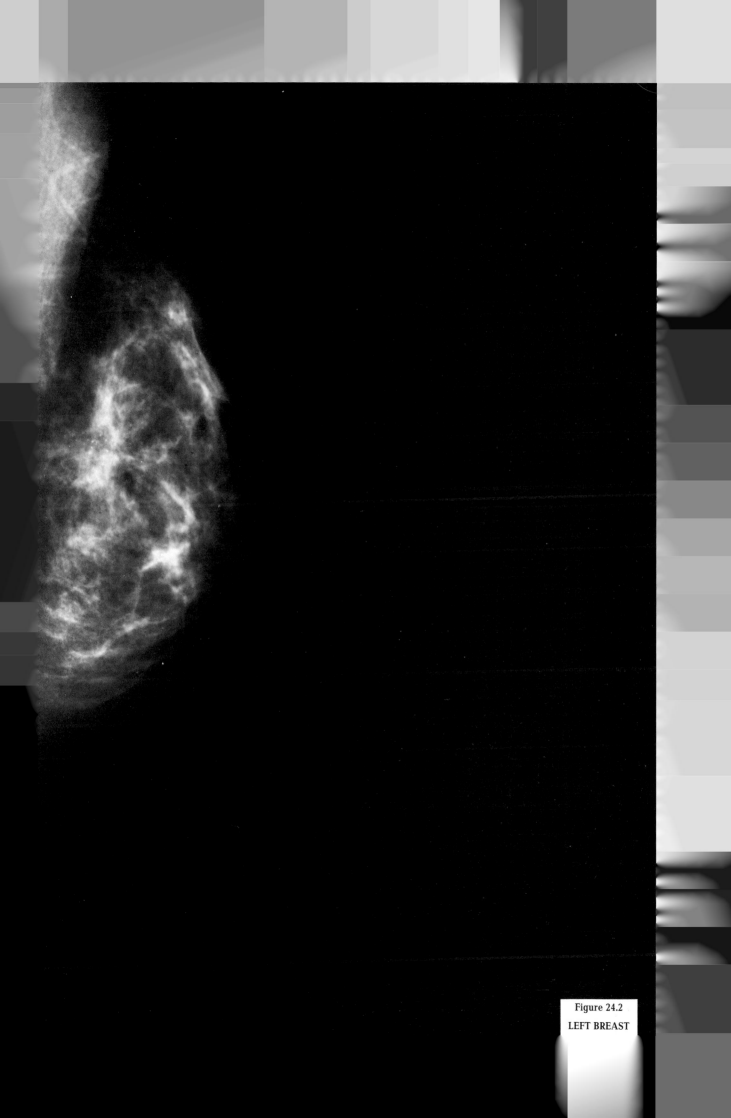

Figure 24.2
LEFT BREAST

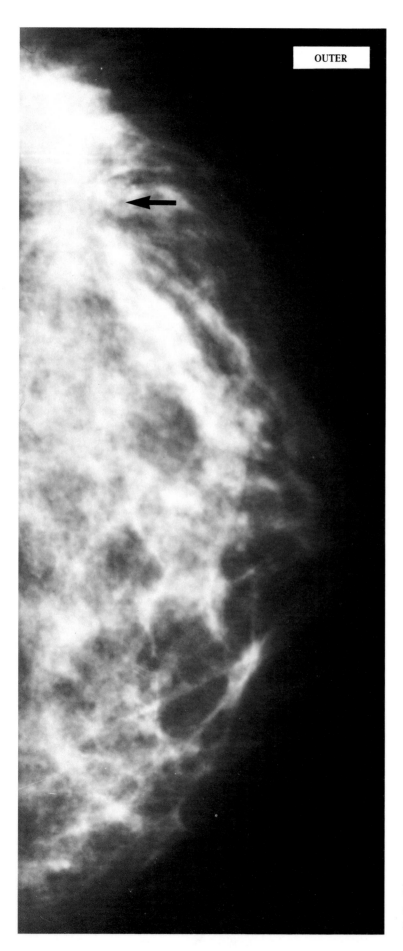

OUTER

Figure 24.3

Cephalocaudal view shows architectural
distortion (arrow) in the outer hemisphere.

Findings

An architectural distortion with spiculation and microcalcifications (J6) is present in the left breast.

Discussion

The cephalocaudal view *(Figure 24.3)* shows that the spiculated lesion (arrow) is in the outer hemisphere. Because of the relatively radiolucent center of the lesion, a benign condition, such as sclerosing adenosis, was suspected. A biopsy scar could also have this appearance, but there was no history of previous surgery. Because carcinoma could not be excluded with certainty, a biopsy was performed. The pathology specimen showed a radial scar *(Figures 24.4 and 24.5)*.

Radial scar is a benign lesion that is said to occur at the rate of approximately 1 in 1000 screening mammograms.[143] Synonyms for radial scar include infiltrating epitheliosis, benign sclerosing ductal proliferation, and nonencapsulated sclerosing lesion.[5,6] This condition is not related to previous surgery and lies within the spectrum of fibrocystic changes. It is not a precursor to carcinoma. It has been hypothesized that the lesion represents an area of proliferative adenosis, the center of which is undergoing atrophy with fibrosis and retraction of surrounding tissue. On mammography, it is a stellate lesion, manifested by retraction and distortion of breast tissues. Round calcifications are present in over 60 percent of cases.[6] Radial scars are usually not palpable. Although the radiolucent center of the lesion in mammograms is a clue to the correct diagnosis, a biopsy is necessary to rule out malignancy with certainty.[5]

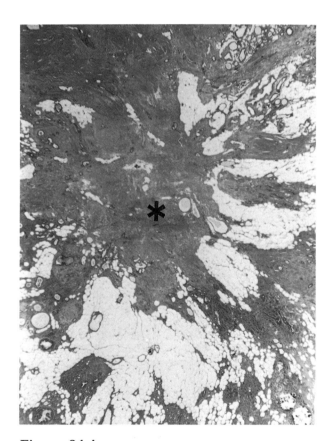

Figure 24.4

Low-power histologic section. The center of the lesion (asterisk) contains fibrosis encasing ducts, lobules and fat. The ducts in the periphery are arranged in a characteristic radial fashion with retraction towards the center. **Diagnosis**: Radial scar.

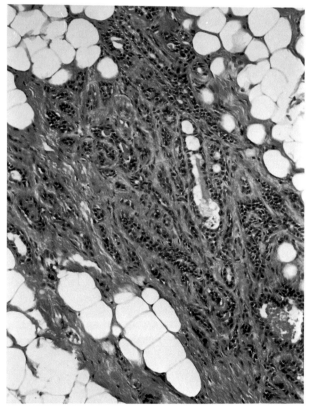

Figure 24.5

High-power. Peripheral region of adenosis with proliferation of epithelial cells and stromal fibrosis.

Case 25

This 50-year-old woman was referred for screening mammography.

Films: Right *(Figure 25.1)* and left *(Figure 25.2)* cephalocaudal mammograms.

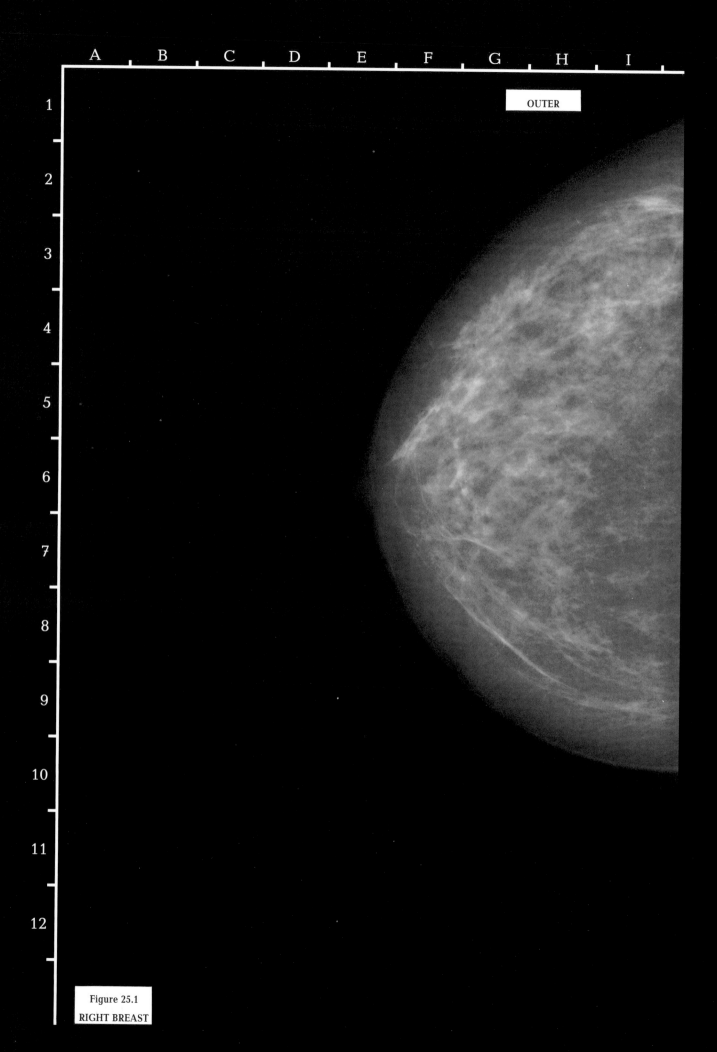

OUTER

Figure 25.1
RIGHT BREAST

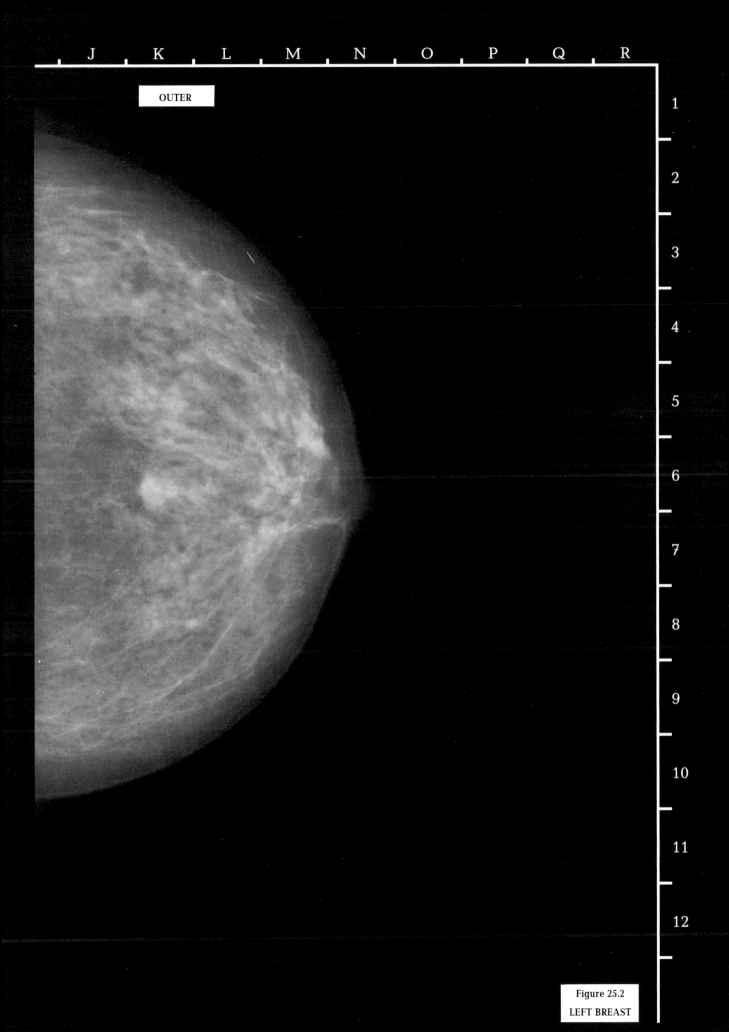

OUTER

J K L M N O P Q R

1 2 3 4 5 6 7 8 9 10 11 12

Figure 25.2
LEFT BREAST

Findings

The ducts are prominent in both breasts. The left breast contains a 1 cm density with irregular borders (K6).

Discussion

The lesion was not evident on a screening mammogram performed 1 year earlier *(Figure 25.3 and Figure 25.4)*. A biopsy was recommended, and revealed infiltrating ductal carcinoma.

The case illustrates the usefulness of regular mammography screening in the detection of breast cancer.[94] In the US, the Breast Cancer Detection Demonstration Project showed an initial prevalence of 7 cancers per 1000 women screened, and an annual incidence of 3 per 1000.[11] Although both physical examination and mammography were used, 42 percent of these cancers were detected only by mammography, and 7 percent only by physical examination. In the

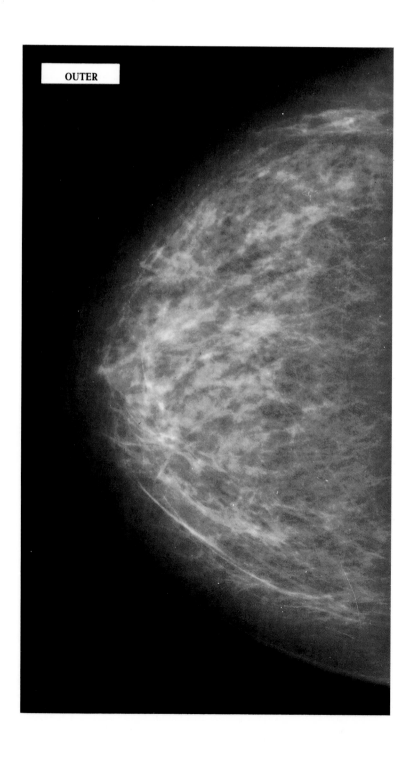

Swedish 2-county study, after 7 years, screening mammography had yielded a 31 percent reduction in mortality and a 25 percent reduction in Stage II or more advanced cancers compared to the non-screened control group.[144] Guidelines for screening mammography are controversial. A consensus of professional medical societies in the US including the American Cancer Society, American College of Radiology and National Cancer Institute recommends mammograms every 1–2 years for women aged 40–49 and annually for women aged 50 and older.[4]

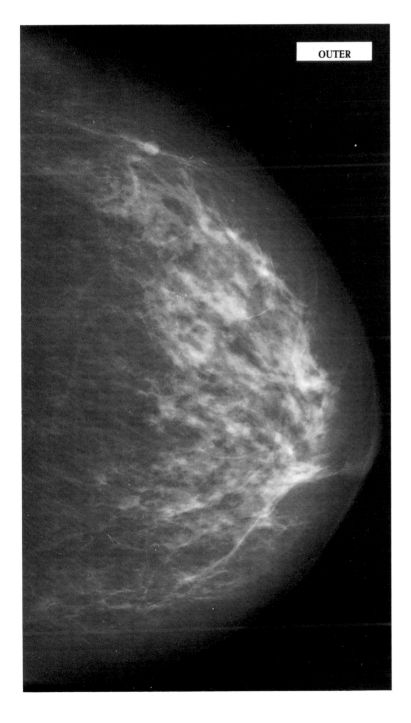

OUTER

Figure 25.3 and 25.4

Right and left cephalocaudal mammograms 1 year previously.

Case 26

A 34-year-old woman had a burning sensation and redness of the left breast.

Films: Right *(Figure 26.1)* and left *(Figure 26.2)* mediolateral oblique mammograms.

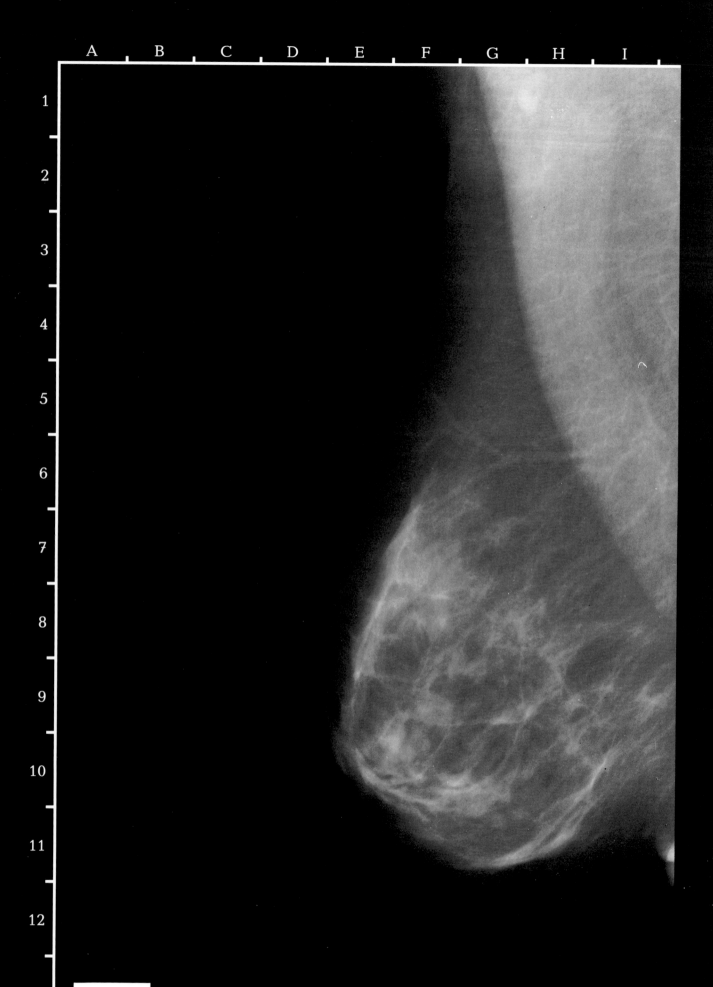

Figure 26.1
RIGHT BREAST

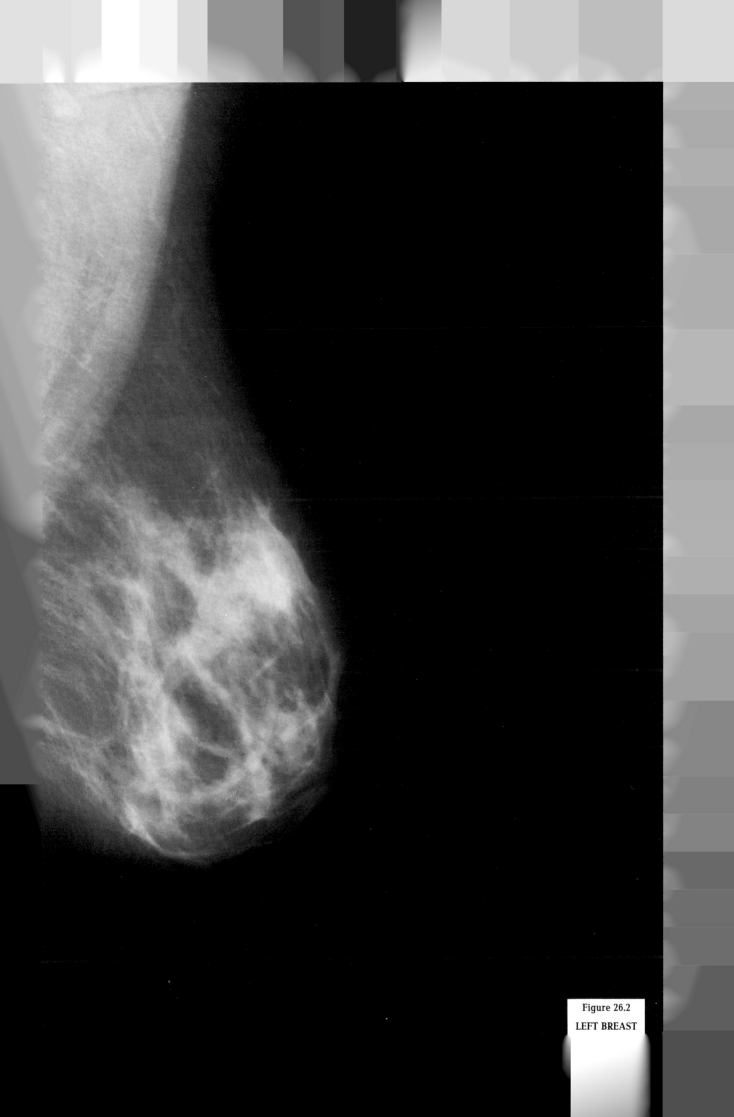

Figure 26.2
LEFT BREAST

Findings

An area of bilaterally asymmetric increased parenchymal density (L7) is present in the left breast.

Discussion

The asymmetric density is confirmed in the cephalocaudal projections *(Figures 26.3 and 26.4)*, and architectural distortion is visible at its margins. No abnormalities were found on physical examination. Biopsy of the density revealed intraductal carcinoma *(Figure 26.5)*.

Asymmetry of parenchymal density may result from normal variations in the involution of breast parenchyma, previous biopsy, or fibrocystic changes. Asymmetry may also be associated with breast carcinoma.[96] In a review of 8408 mammograms, there were 221 (3 percent) with asymmetric parenchymal tissue without architectural

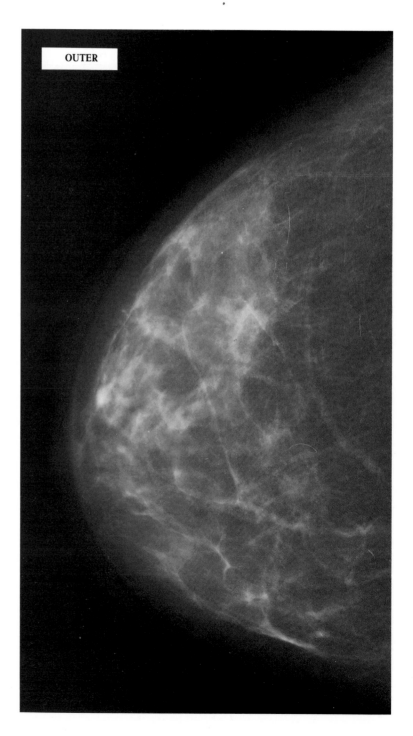

Figure 26.3

Cephalocaudal view of right breast shows no abnormalities.

distortion.[79] Of the 20 patients who underwent biopsy for clinical findings, 3 had carcinomas, all of which were manifested by a palpable abnormality. Mammographic follow-up of the remaining 201 patients for 36–42 months failed to show evidence of breast carcinoma. Therefore, parenchymal asymmetry alone is an insufficient cause for biopsy. To warrant a biopsy in an asymptomatic patient, the asymmetry should be associated with an architectural distortion.

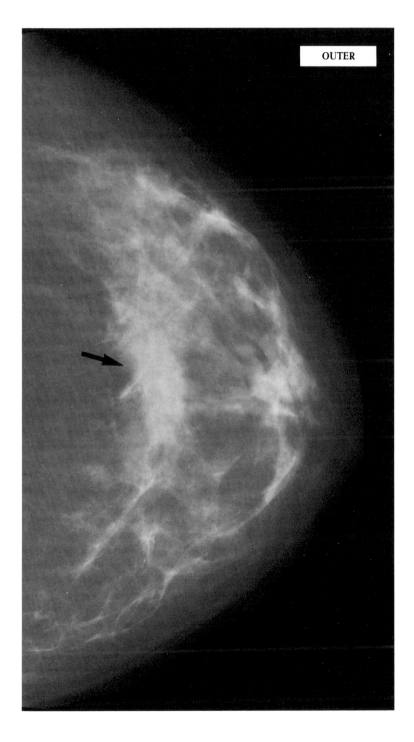

OUTER

Figure 26.4

Cephalocaudal view of left breast reveals area of asymmetry (arrow).

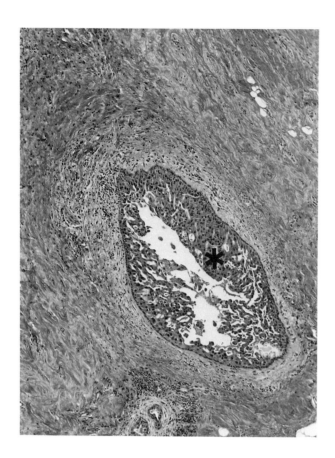

Figure 26.5

Low-power histologic section. Malignant intraductal epithelial cells encroach on and partially obliterate the duct lumen (asterisk). There is marked periductal fibrosis. **Diagnosis**: intraductal carcinoma.

Case 27

This 79-year-old woman had a lump in the right breast.

Films: Right *(Figure 27.1)* and left *(Figure 27.2)* mediolateral oblique mammograms.

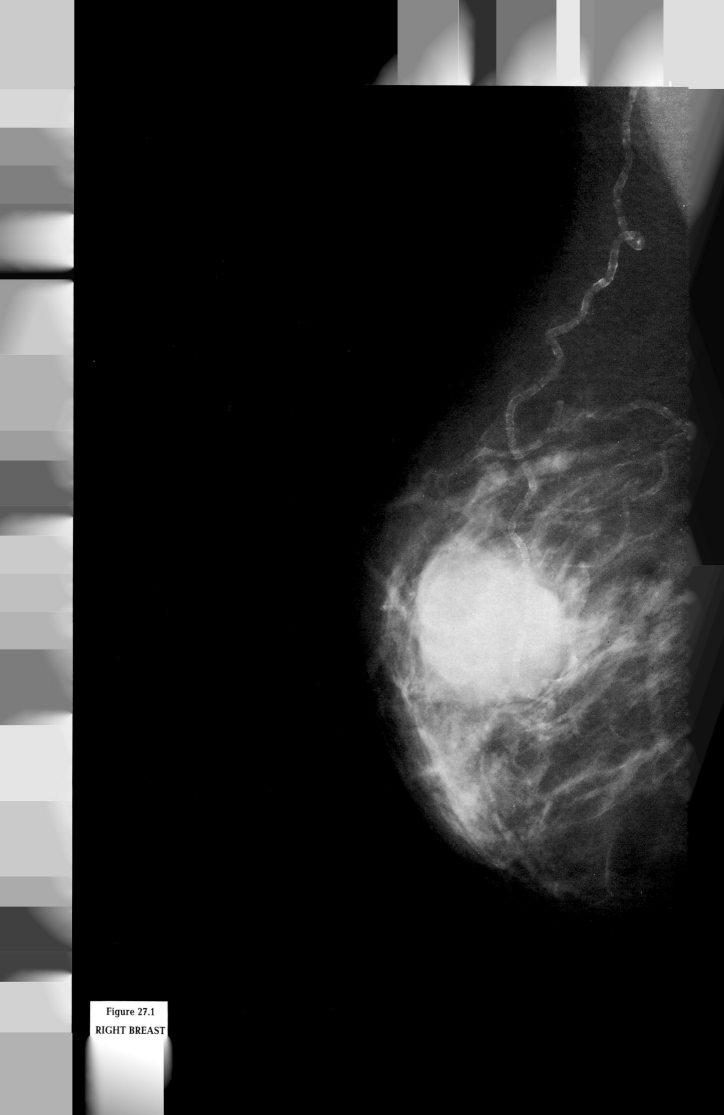

Figure 27.1
RIGHT BREAST

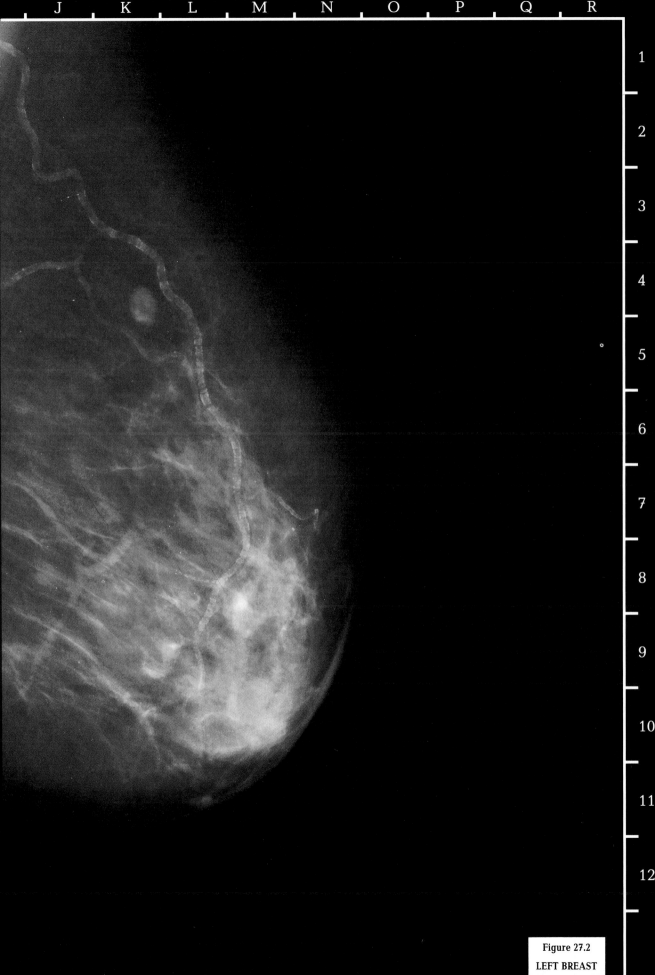

Figure 27.2
LEFT BREAST

Findings

There is a 3.5 cm mass (G8) in the right breast. There is a 1 cm oval density (K4) in the upper hemisphere of the left breast. Arterial calcifications are seen bilaterally. Large veins are present on the right.

Discussion

Calcifications in the walls of arteries typically show a 'railroad track' pattern and are a common finding, especially in older patients.[133] The oval density in the left breast is well circumscribed and has a radiolucent center *(Figure 27.3)*, typical of a benign intramammary lymph node.[38] The palpable mass in the right breast is dense and relatively well circumscribed. Sonography revealed that it was solid, and biopsy was recommended. Pathology disclosed an infiltrating papillary carcinoma *(Figure 27.4 and Figure 27.5)*.

Papillary carcinoma is uncommon, making up only about 2 percent of all cases of breast carcinoma.[72] The cancer grows in a papillary form within dilated ducts and cysts. It has a tendency to occur in the larger collecting ducts of the central part of the breast, and may present with nipple discharge, often bloody.[54,80] Mammographically, it tends to have a more well-defined margin than infiltrating ductal carcinoma,[123] and since it rarely metastasizes it has a better prognosis.[46]

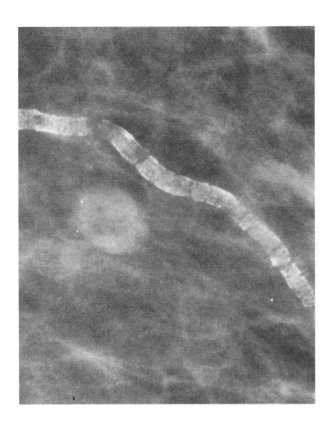

Figure 27.3

Close-up of left breast mass shows well-circumscribed margin and lucent center. Adjacent to the mass is a calcified artery.

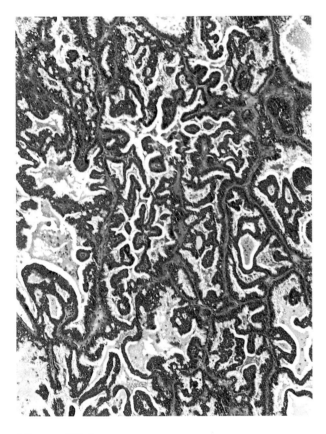

Figure 27.4

Low-power histologic section of right breast mass. Complex papillary proliferations are seen within dilated ducts. **Diagnosis**: Papillary carcinoma.

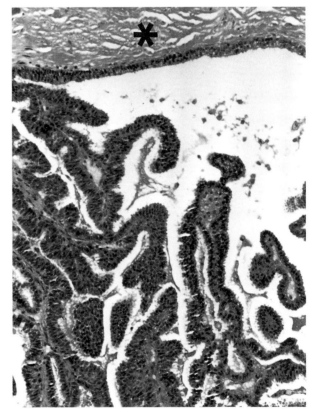

Figure 27.5

Outer fibrous wall (asterisk) produces smooth margin seen in the mammogram.

Case 28

This 52-year-old woman has a family history of breast cancer in her mother and sister. She was referred because of a mammographic abnormality in the right breast.

Films: Right *(Figure 28.1)* and left *(Figure 28.2)* mediolateral mammograms.

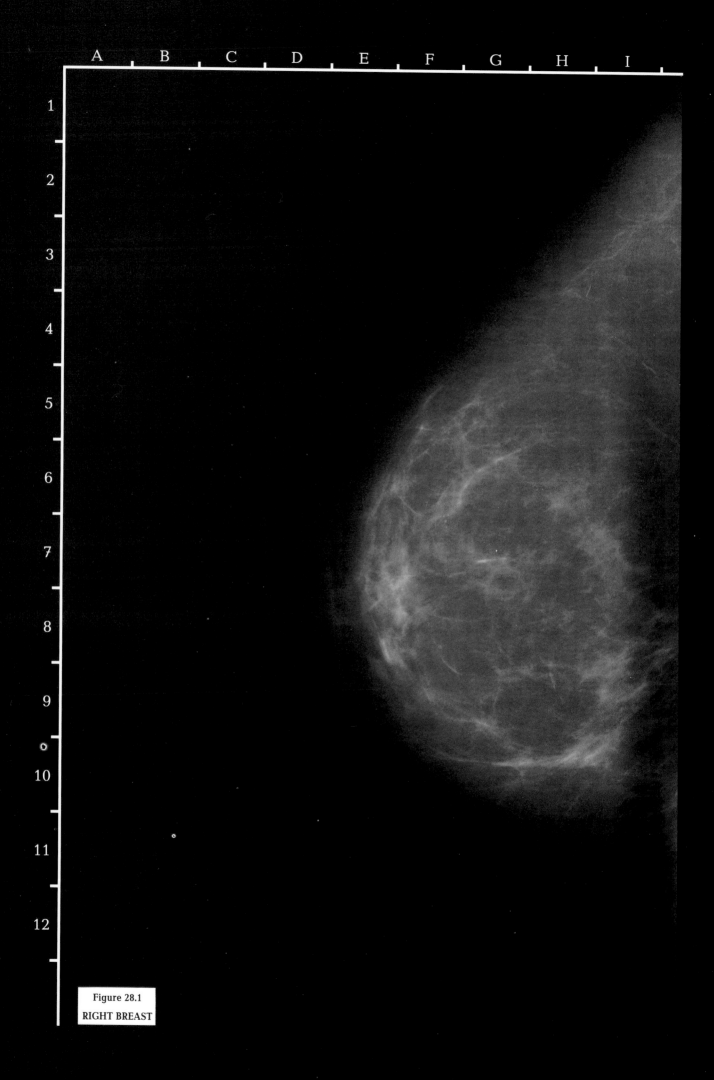

Figure 28.1
RIGHT BREAST

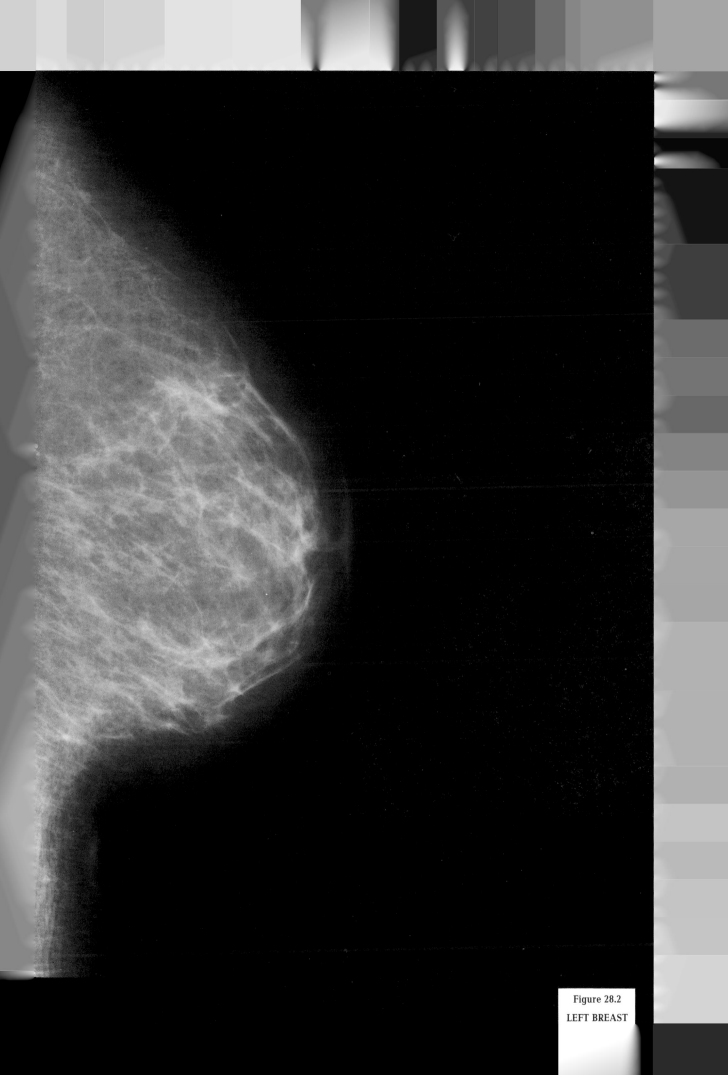

Figure 28.2
LEFT BREAST

Findings

There are small groups of calcifications in the right (F7) and left (J6) breasts.

Discussion

The calcifications in the left breast have the typical appearance of dermal deposits: they are few in number, spherical, of low density and some have lucent centers. On the right, the calcifications are also few in number and low in density, but their dermal origin is not as certain because of their irregular shape. In the cephalocaudal view, although the calcifications are difficult to see, they are located near the medial surface of the breast (Figure 28.3). Because of the strong family history of breast carcinoma, it was important to prove the dermal location of the calcifications on the right.

A radiopaque marker was placed on the medial surface of the right breast at the estimated site of the calcifications.[17] A mediolateral mammogram verified that the marker was at the site of the calcifications (Figure 28.4). With the marker overlying the calcifications, it will maintain its close proximity to the calcifications in any subsequent projection if the calcifications are in the skin.[77] Likewise, a mammogram performed tangential to the marker will show the intradermal location of the calcifications (Figure 28.5).

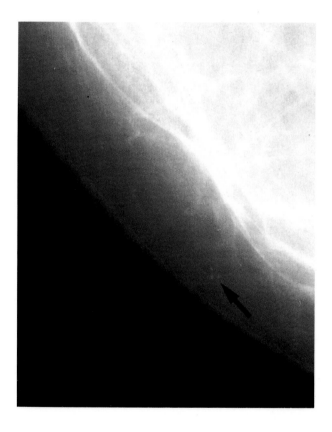

Figure 28.3

Close-up of right cephalocaudal mammogram shows calcifications (arrow) near medial skin surface.

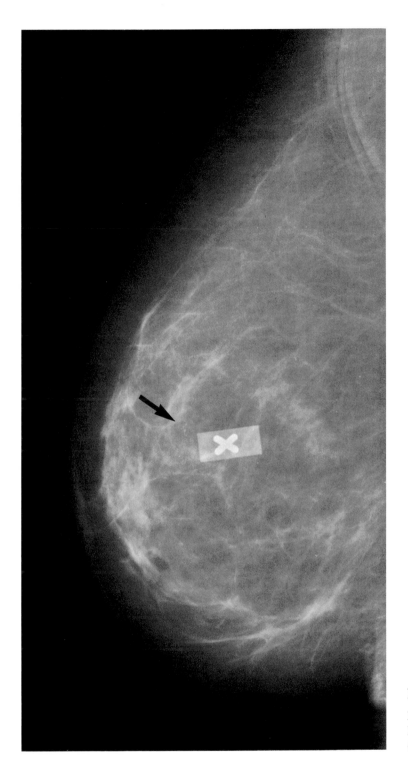

Figure 28.4

Mediolateral view of right breast.
Radiopaque marker is at the site of the
calcifications (arrow).

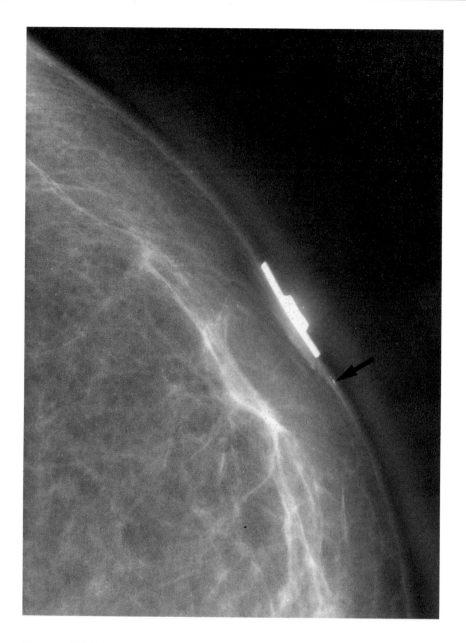

Figure 28.5

View tangential to radiopaque marker depicts calcifications (arrow) in the skin.

Case 29

This 56-year-old woman was asymptomatic.

***Films*:** Right *(Figure 29.1)* and left *(Figure 29.2)* mediolateral mammograms.

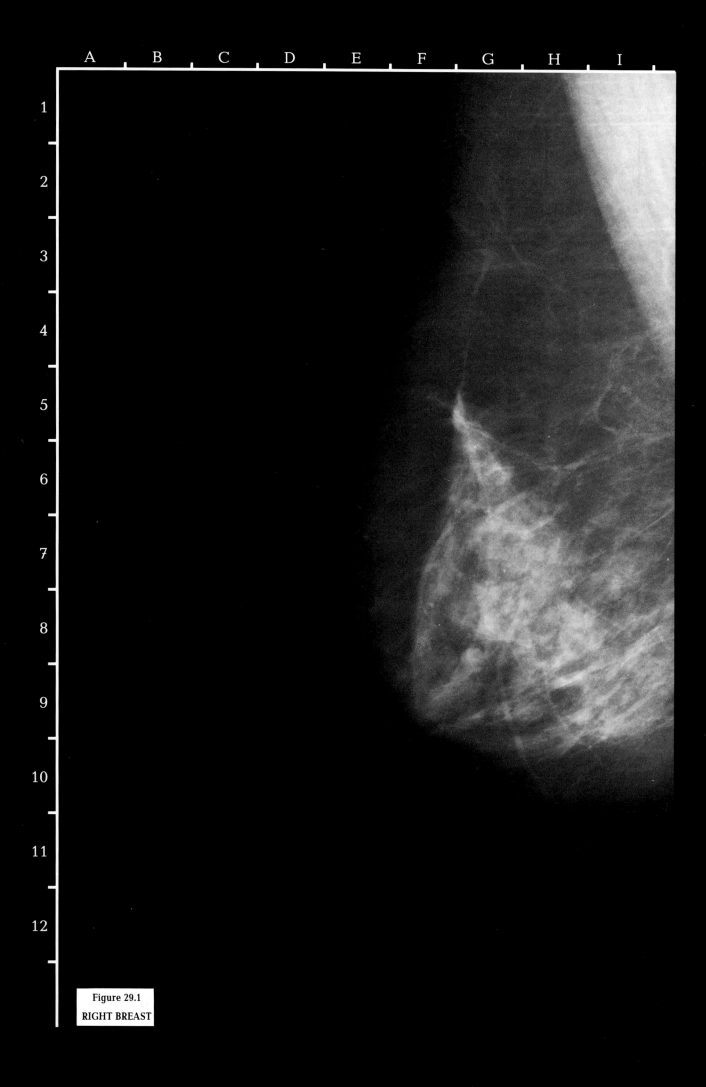

Figure 29.1
RIGHT BREAST

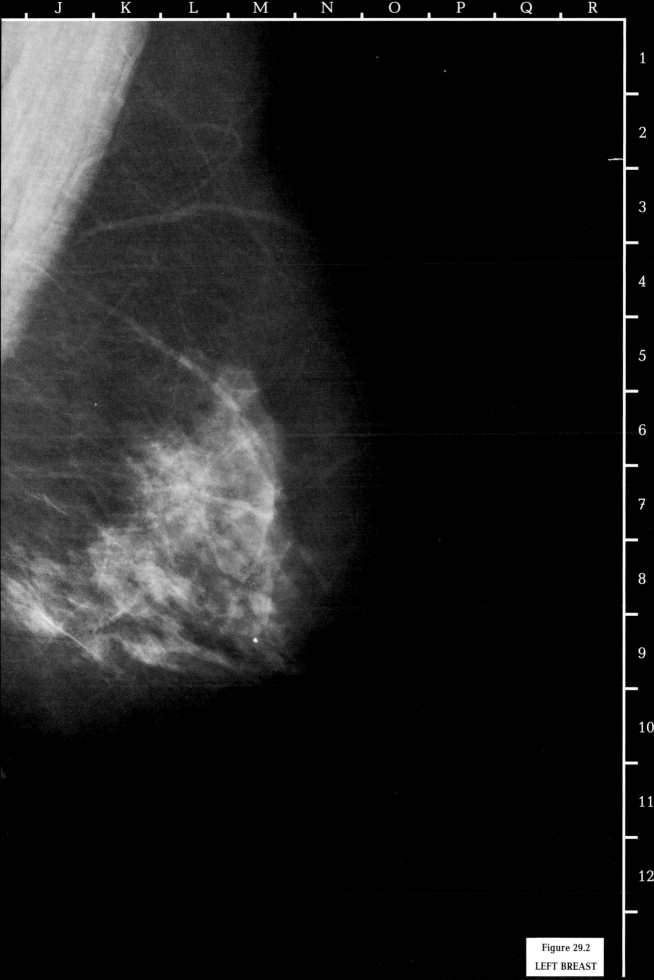

J K L M N O P Q R

1
2
3
4
5
6
7
8
9
10
11
12

Figure 29.2
LEFT BREAST

Findings

There is an architectural distortion (F5) in the upper hemisphere of the right breast. Benign-appearing scattered calcifications are present bilaterally.

Discussion

The suspicious architectural distortion was confirmed by mediolateral and cephalocaudal magnification views *(Figures 29.3 and 29.4)*. The lesion was localized with a hookwire and removed *(Figure 29.5)*. Histologic examination revealed infiltrating ductal carcinoma *(Figure 29.6)*.

This case is an example of architectural distortion resulting from a desmoplastic reaction to infiltrating ductal carcinoma. The distortion is due to radiating strands projecting from a shrinking process of fibrosis. These strands may produce a stellate appearance as they radiate from a central mass. Sometimes the mass is not evident and the radiographic abnormality is dominated, as in this case, by the retracted tissue strands themselves.[5]

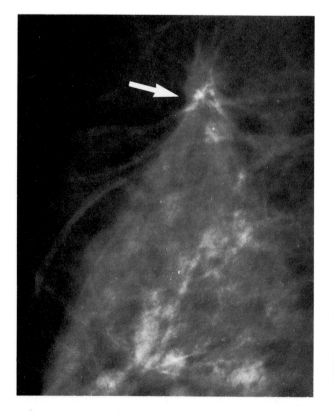

Figure 29.3

Right mediolateral magnification view verifies the architectural distortion (arrow).

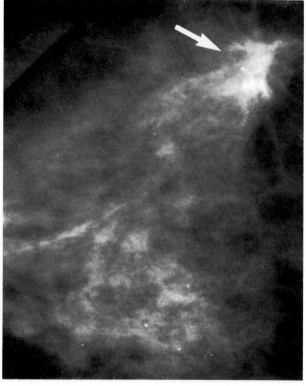

Figure 29.4

Cephalocaudal magnification view shows the suspicious lesion (arrow).

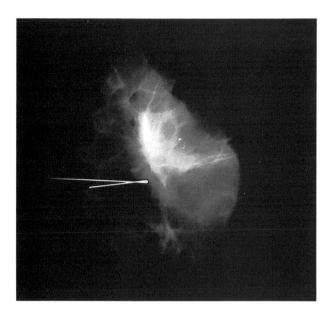

Figure 29.5

Specimen radiograph confirms that the irregular density has been excised and includes the tip of the hookwire.

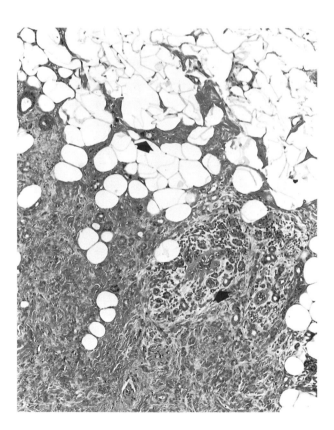

Figure 29.6

Low-power histologic section. Irregular neoplastic glands (arrows) infiltrate adjacent lobules and adipose tissue.

Case 30

This 31-year-old woman had a mass in the upper–outer quadrant of the left breast, near the axilla.

Films: Right *(Figure 30.1)* and left *(Figure 30.2)* mediolateral oblique views, and right *(Figure 30.3)* and left *(Figure 30.4)* cephalocaudal views.

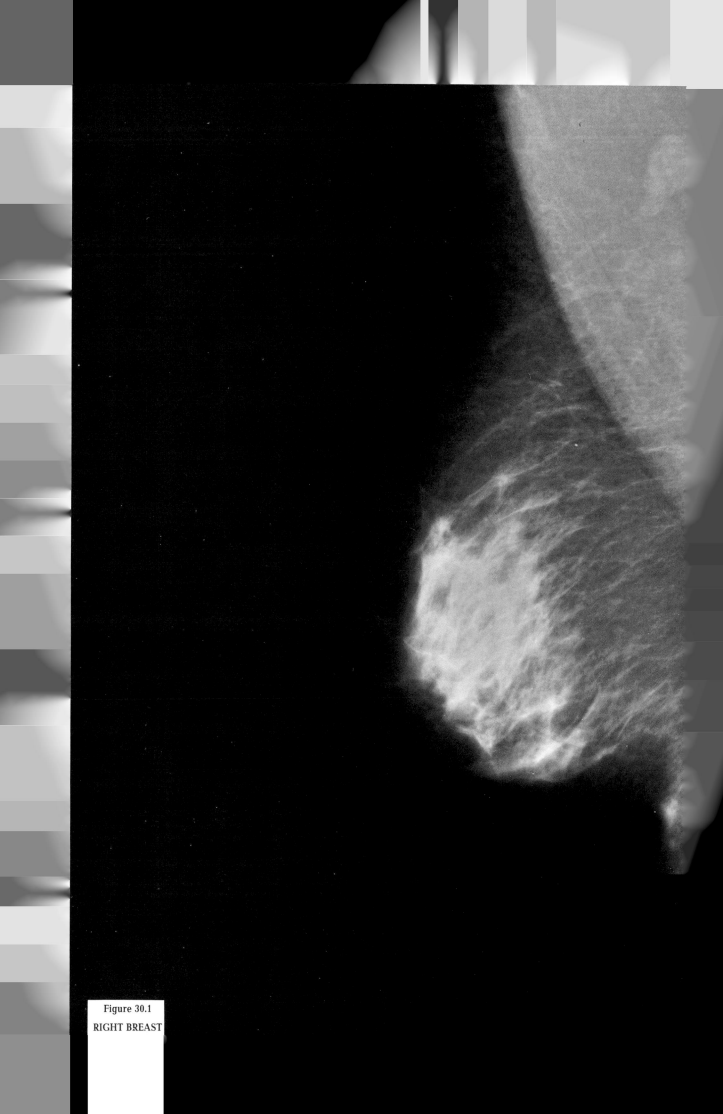

Figure 30.1
RIGHT BREAST

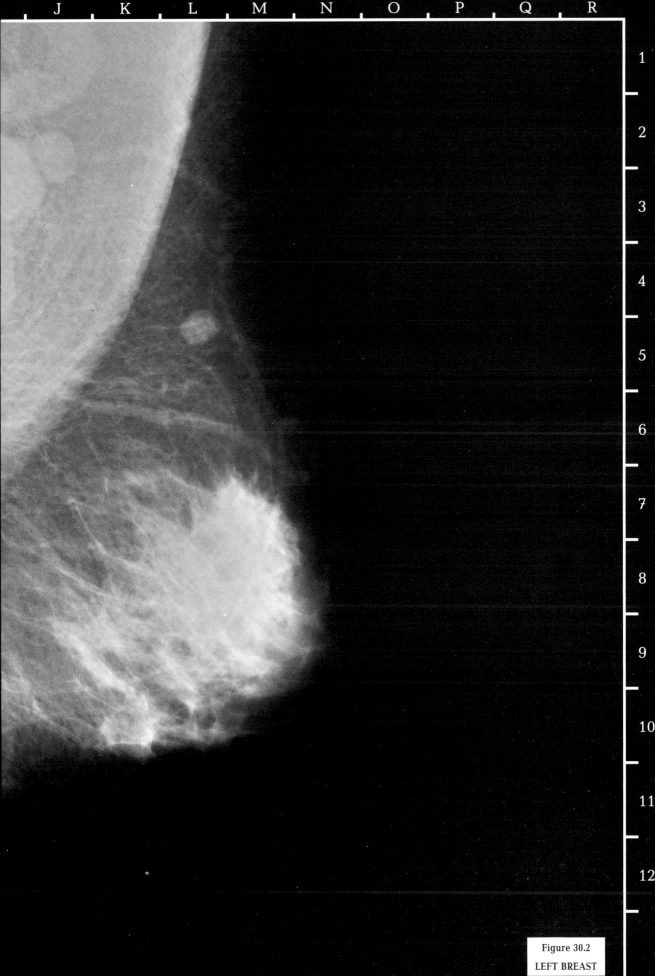

Figure 30.2
LEFT BREAST

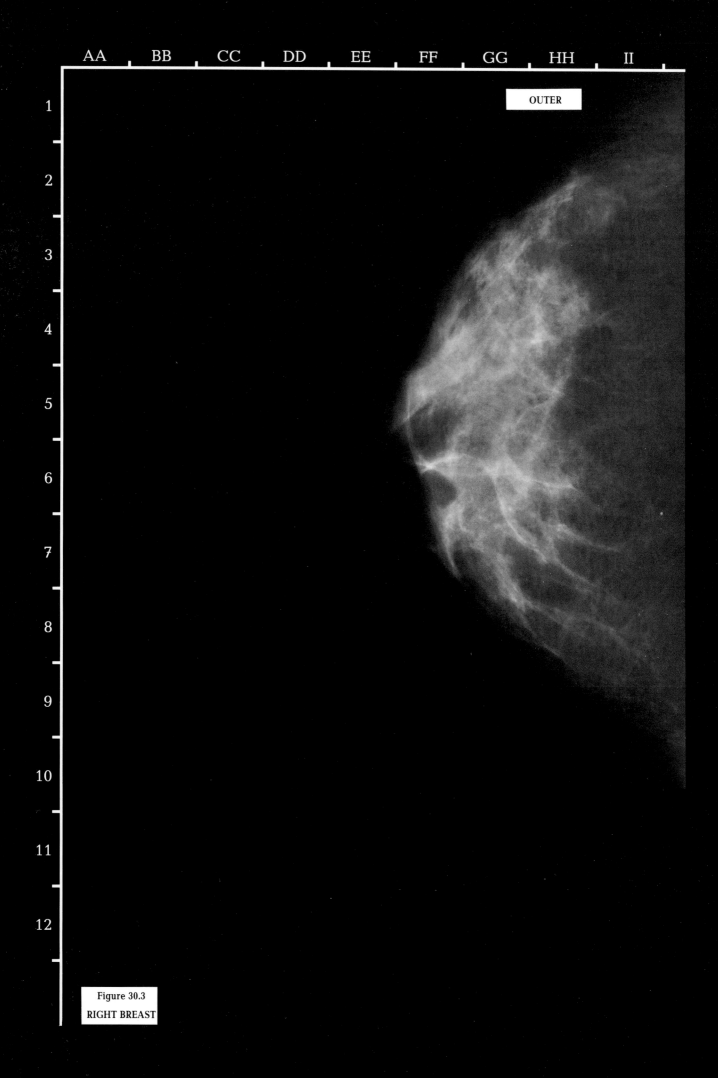

AA　　BB　　CC　　DD　　EE　　FF　　GG　　HH　　II

OUTER

1
2
3
4
5
6
7
8
9
10
11
12

Figure 30.3
RIGHT BREAST

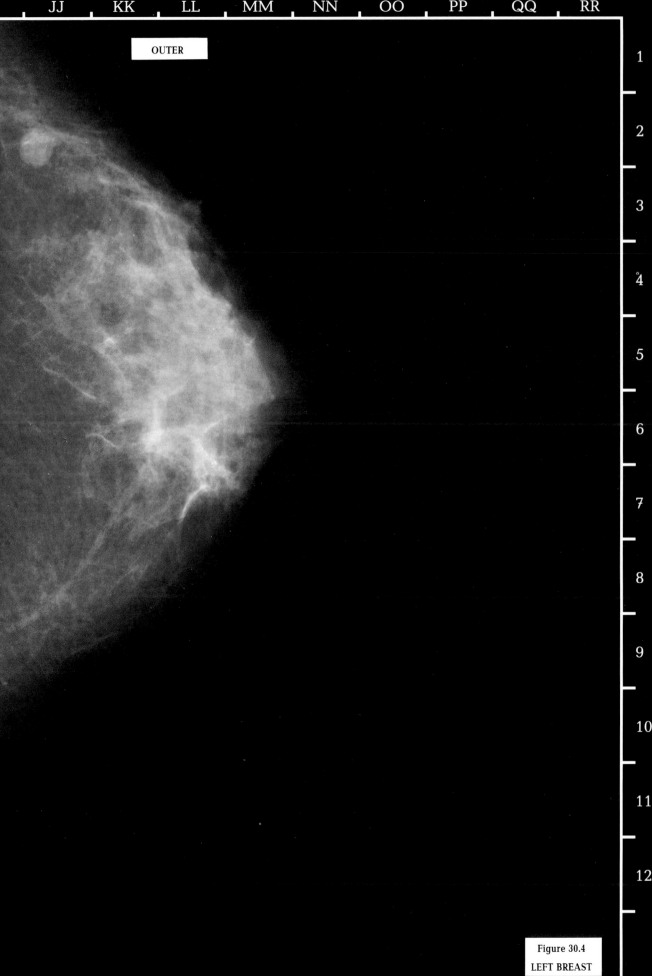

JJ   KK   LL   MM   NN   OO   PP   QQ   RR

OUTER

1   2   3   4   5   6   7   8   9   10   11   12

Figure 30.4
LEFT BREAST

Findings

A well-circumscribed 1 cm nodule is present in the upper–outer quadrant of the left breast (L5), (JJ2). Large, dense lymph nodes are seen in both axillae and are more prominent on the left. A small group of subareolar calcifications is depicted in the cephalocaudal view (LL6), but they are not visualized in the mediolateral oblique view.

Discussion

In the mediolateral view *(Figure 30.5)* the microcalcifications are better depicted, and the palpable mass manifests a 'halo sign'. The halo sign refers to a narrow radiolucent ring—a negative Mach effect—seen around the periphery of a mass in film-screen mammograms. This finding usually implies a benign tumor,[143] although a circumferential or partial halo sign sometimes accompanies a well-circumscribed carcinoma.[142] Sonography *(Figure 30.6)* indicated that the mass was solid, highly echogenic and well circumscribed—features suggestive but not diagnostic of a fibroadenoma or intramammary lymph node. A biopsy of the mass was performed. Histologic examination *(Figure 30.7)* and immunohistochemical evaluation showed that the mass was an intramammary lymph node that contained metastatic carcinoma. Subsequent mastectomy revealed underlying infiltrating lobular carcinoma, manifested in the mammograms only by the small cluster of calcifications.

Metastatic disease to intramammary lymph nodes from breast cancer may be recognized mammographically. The affected nodes tend to be enlarged (1 cm or greater), homogeneous, well circumscribed and lacking the central lucency characteristic of benign intramammary lymph nodes.[88] Comparison with previous mammograms may show progressive enlargement of the node. An enlarged or enlarging intramammary lymph node mandates careful search of the mammogram for signs of an underlying primary malignancy.

Histologic examination of the axillary lymph nodes confirmed the presence of metastatic disease. Axillary nodes are commonly seen in mediolateral oblique views of the breast. Normal axillary nodes are well defined, medium-to-low in density and usually less than 1.5 cm in diameter.[69] A lucent center or notch representing fat in the hilum is often seen in benign nodes. Coarse calcification may be seen in nodes affected by granulomatous disease. Enlarged nodes may be present in rheumatoid arthritis. Malignant involvement may occur with lymphoma or metastases from carcinoma of the breast or from extramammary primaries. Malignant axillary nodes tend to be enlarged and dense. When the criteria for abnormality include a nonfatty node with a size over 2.5 cm, the true-positive rate for predicting axillary nodal metastases is 100 percent and the false-negative rate is 41 percent.[70]

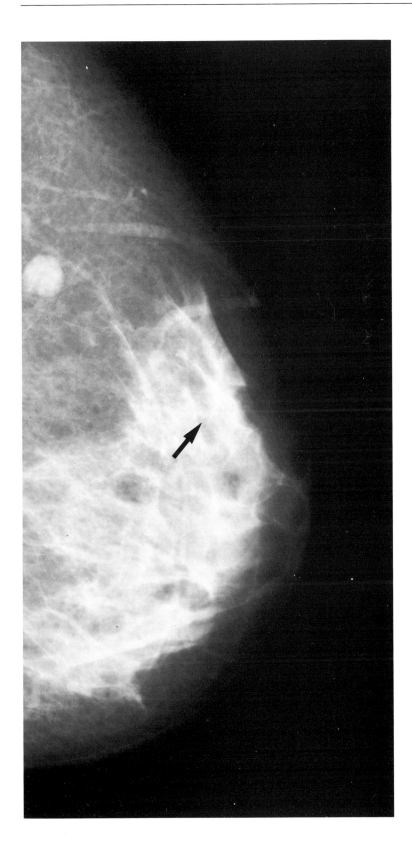

Figure 30.5

Lateral view of the left breast. The mass in the upper hemisphere is well circumscribed and demonstrates a peripheral 'halo'. The calcifications (barely visible in region of arrow) are located 2.5 cm above the nipple.

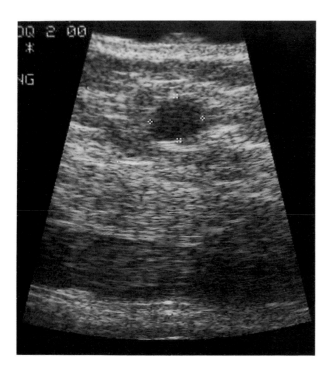

Figure 30.6

Sonogram of palpable mass. The mass is well circumscribed, contains multiple echoes distributed evenly throughout and shows no effect on the echoes posterior to it.

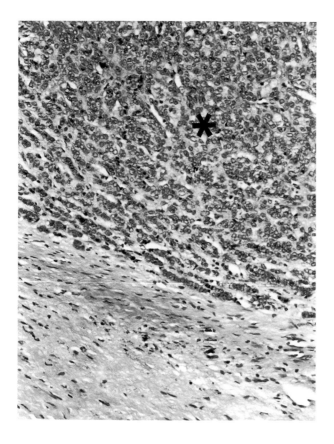

Figure 30.7

High-power histologic section of left intramammary node. There are sheets of poorly differentiated malignant cells (asterisk) with complete effacement of the nodal architecture. Tumor was confined to the node, explaining the well-defined mammographic margins. **Diagnosis**: Lobular carcinoma, metastatic to intramammary lymph node.

Case 31

This 39-year-old asymptomatic woman was referred because of an abnormal screening mammogram.

Films: Right *(Figure 31.1)* and left *(Figure 31.2)* mediolateral oblique mammograms.

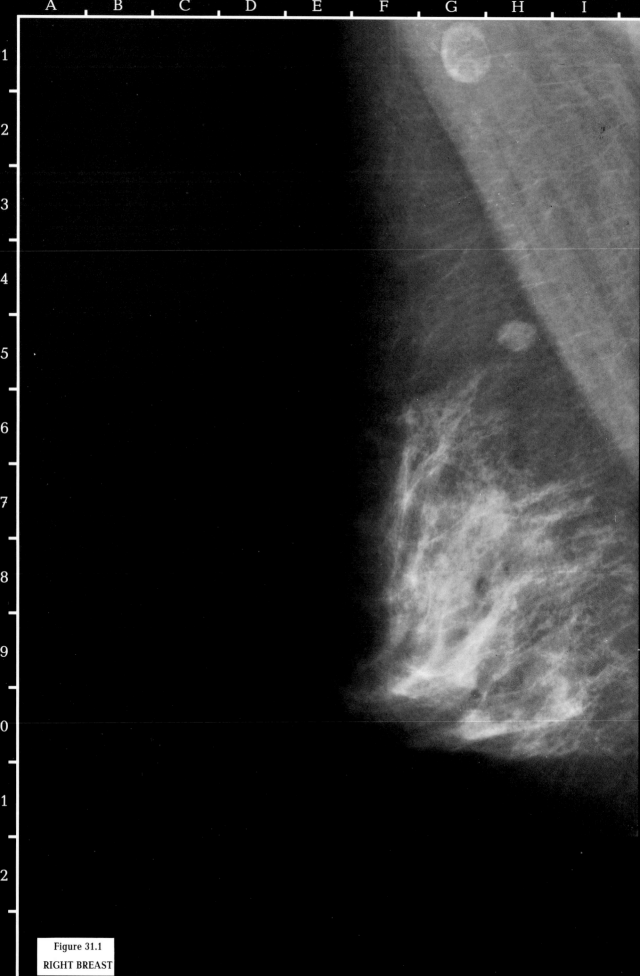

Figure 31.1
RIGHT BREAST

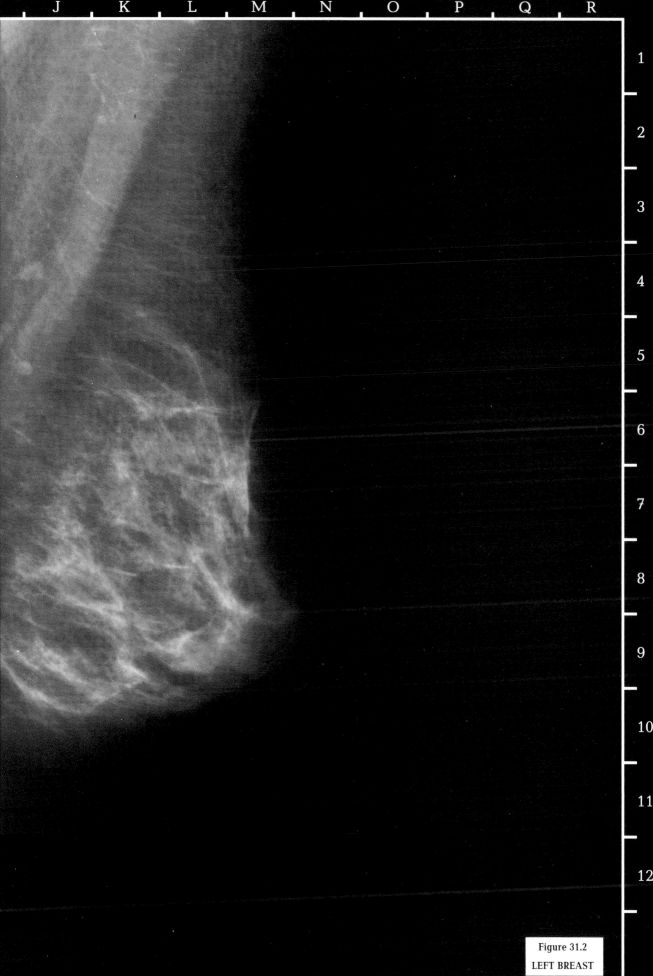

J K L M N O P Q R

1
2
3
4
5
6
7
8
9
10
11
12

Figure 31.2
LEFT BREAST

Findings

In the right breast, there is an axillary lymph node with a radiolucent center (G1), and a 1 cm mass (H5) in the upper hemisphere, anterior to the pectoral muscle.

Several small (5 mm or less), well-defined intra-mammary densities are present in the upper hemisphere of the left breast (J4), (J5).

Discussion

The mass in the right axillary region has typical features of a benign lymph node: it is spherical and has a fat-density center. The multiple nodules in the upper left breast were felt to represent benign lymph nodes.

The mass in the upper hemisphere of the right breast also had features suggesting an intra-mammary lymph node: location in the upper hemisphere and smooth margins. However, its large size compared to the contralateral intra-mammary lymph nodes and the absence of a lucent center were of concern.[38,88] A well-circumscribed carcinoma or a lymph node involved with malignancy could not be ruled out with certainty. This mass had not been imaged in the cephalocaudal view. A 'Cleopatra' view *(Figure 31.3)*, a modified cephalocaudal projection for depicting the tissue in the axillary tail, showed the mass *(Figure 31.4)*. Sonography revealed that the mass was solid. A biopsy was performed.

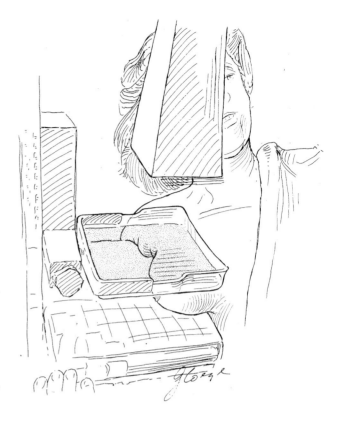

Figure 31.3

Modified, 'Cleopatra', view. The patient is leaning backward, like Cleopatra reclining on her divan, so that the axillary tail of the breast is included in the image.

Histologic examination of the excised specimen revealed a benign intramammary lymph node *(Figure 31.5)*.

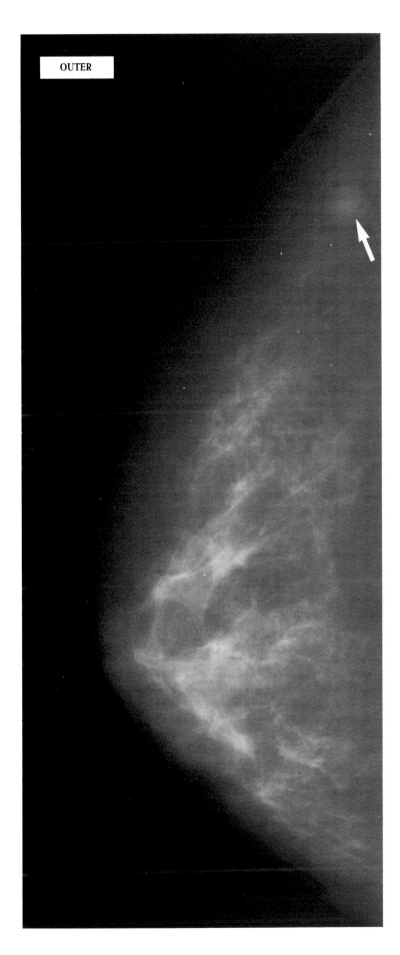

Figure 31.4

Cleopatra view of the right breast. The mass (arrow) is identified in the axillary tail of the breast.

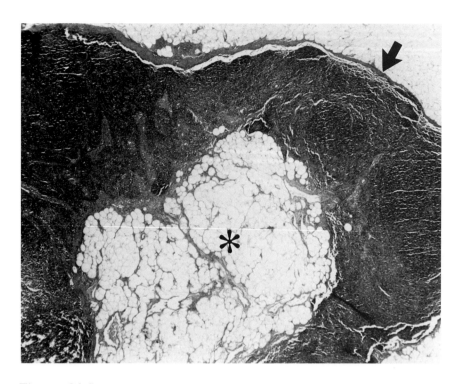

Figure 31.5

Low-power histologic section. Benign lymph node. The capsule (arrow) around the node is responsible for the smooth margin seen in the mammograms. The fat (asterisk) in the hilum of the node was not appreciated in the mammogram, possibly due to the angle of imaging technique.

Case 32

This 70-year-old asymptomatic woman was referred for screening mammography.

Films: Right *(Figure 32.1)* and left *(Figure 32.2)* mediolateral oblique mammograms.

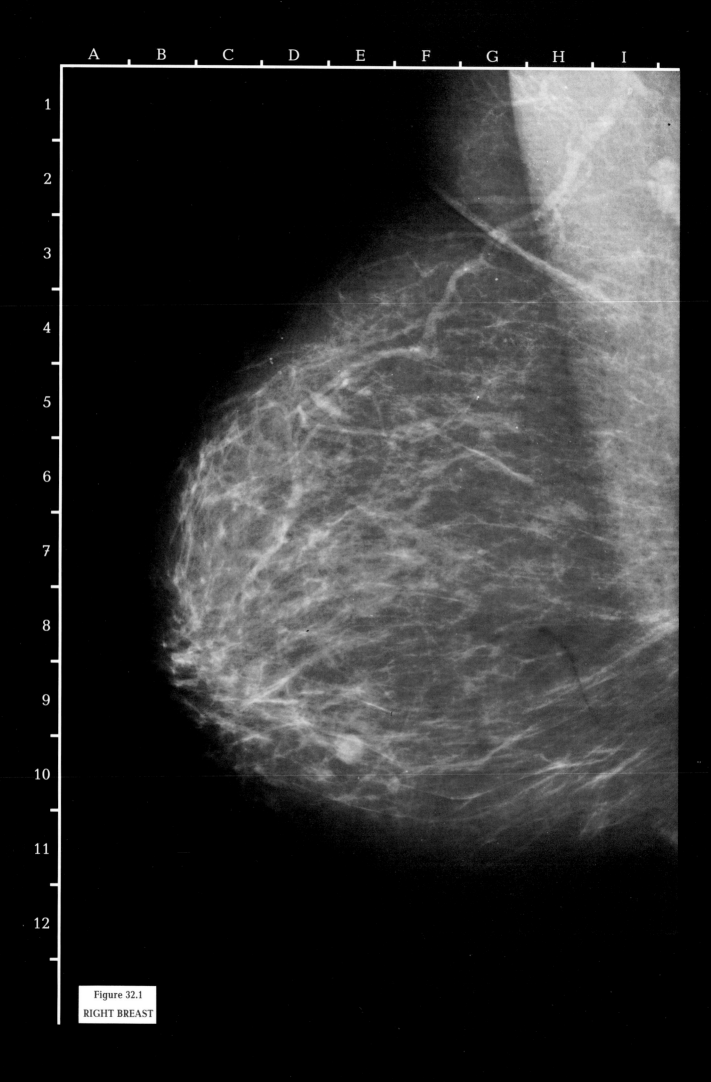

Figure 32.1
RIGHT BREAST

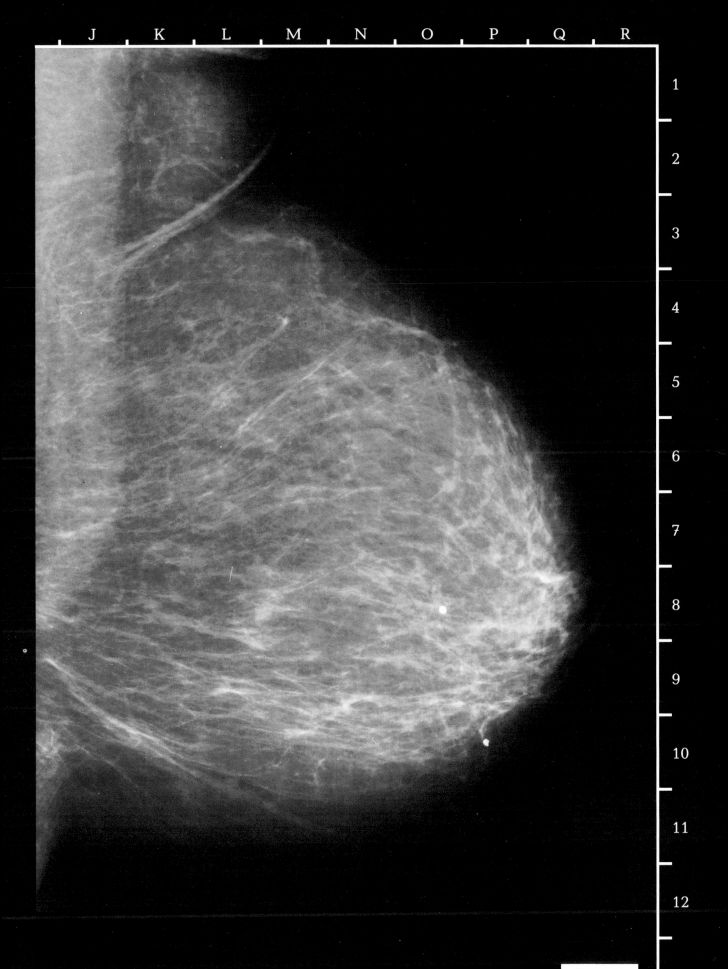

Figure 32.2
LEFT BREAST

Findings

A few coarse, benign calcifications are present bilaterally. There is an 8 mm nodule in the lower hemisphere of the right breast (E10). Part of a lymph node of intermediate density is visualized in the right axilla.

Discussion

The mass was also seen on the cephalocaudal view *(Figure 32.3)*. It was small and relatively well defined, with a surrounding halo. However, the anterior border of the mass is not as well defined as the posterior border. Sonography showed that the mass was solid. Mammograms performed 2 years earlier were retrieved for comparison *(Figure 32.4)*. In the earlier examination, the mass was visible but only 5 mm in diameter. Because of the increase in size, a biopsy was recommended and showed infiltrating ductal carcinoma *(Figure 32.5)*. The axillary lymph nodes were resected and disclosed only sinus histiocytosis, with no evidence of metastasis.

The mass had been assumed to be benign on the earlier examination because of its smooth margins and small size. Indeed, a review of 593 noncalcified masses with smooth margins disclosed that only 2 percent were malignant.[105] However, radiologists cannot make a definitive

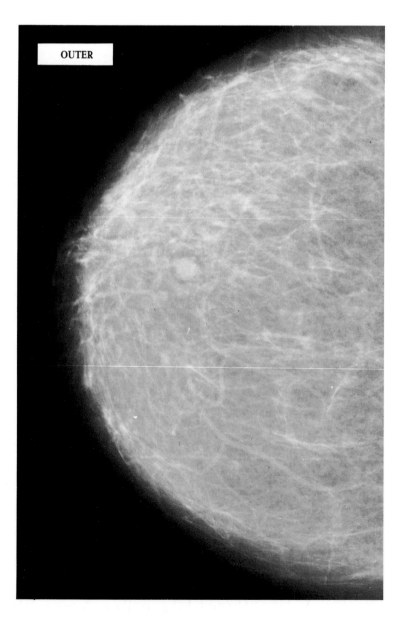

OUTER

Figure 32.3

Right cephalocaudal mammogram. The anterior margin of the 8 mm mass is not as well defined as the posterior margin.

diagnosis of a benign mass on the basis of a single mammographic examination,[21] unless it has the typical 'popcorn calcifications' of fibroadenoma, or the fat content of an intramammary lymph node, galactocele, lipoma or lipofibroadenoma. Therefore, when biopsy of a mass is not undertaken due to its benign mammographic features, follow-up examinations should be performed, first at 6 months and then at yearly intervals for at least 2½ years.[64] Although it could be argued that the mass in the later mammogram should have been biopsied solely due to its irregular anterior margin, recognition that the mass had grown in the interval since the earlier examination clinched the decision. This case also shows the importance of long-term retention of mammograms for comparison with future examinations.

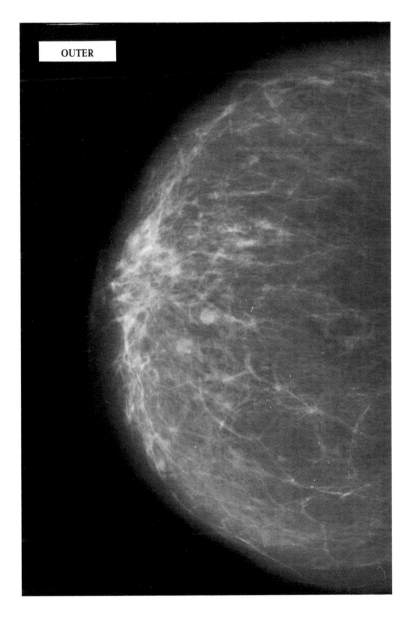

OUTER

Figure 32.4

Right cephalocaudal mammogram performed 2 years earlier. The nodule was 5 mm in size and had smooth margins.

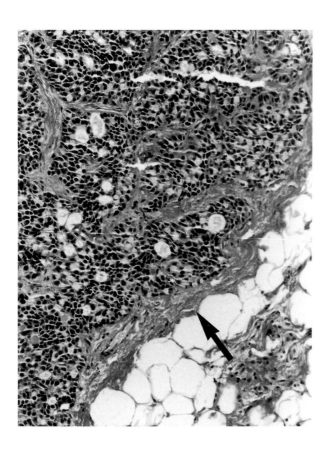

Figure 32.5

Low-power histologic section. There are sheets of malignant ductal epithelium infiltrating a fibrous stroma. The tumor is surrounded by fibrous tissue which has a well-demarcated boundary (arrow) with the adjacent fat. **Diagnosis**: Infiltrating ductal carcinoma.

Case 33

This 30-year-old woman was referred for a mammographic abnormality in the upper–outer quadrant of her right breast.

Films: Mediolateral oblique *(Figure 33.1)* and cephalocaudal *(Figure 33.2)* views of the right breast.

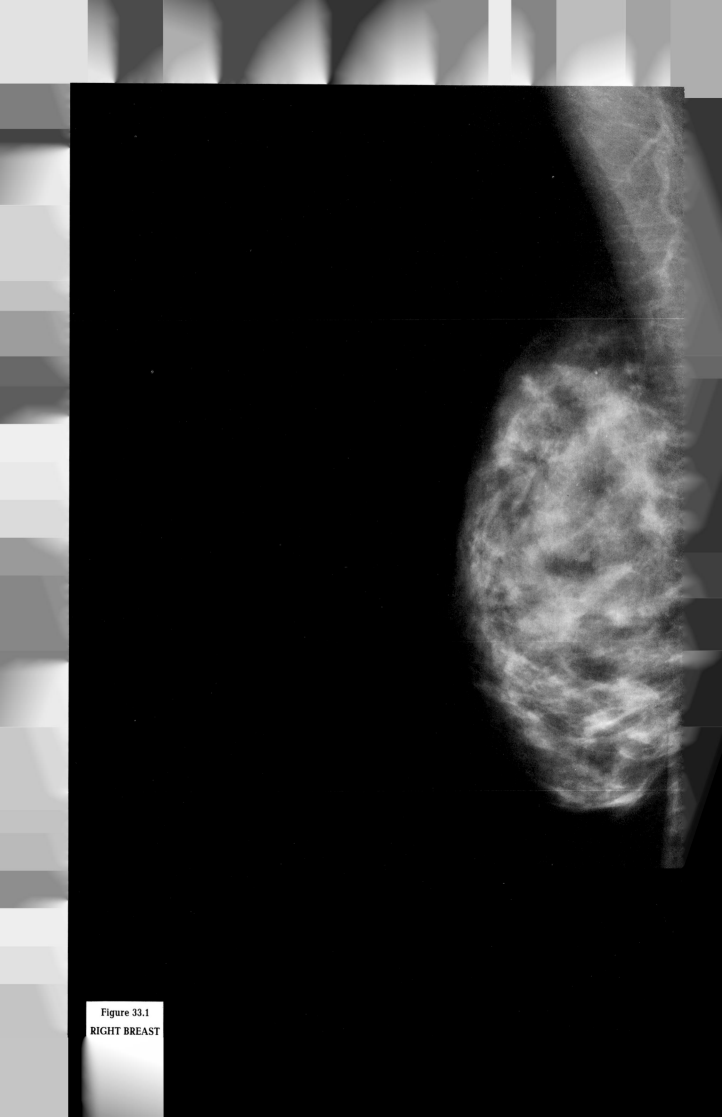

Figure 33.1
RIGHT BREAST

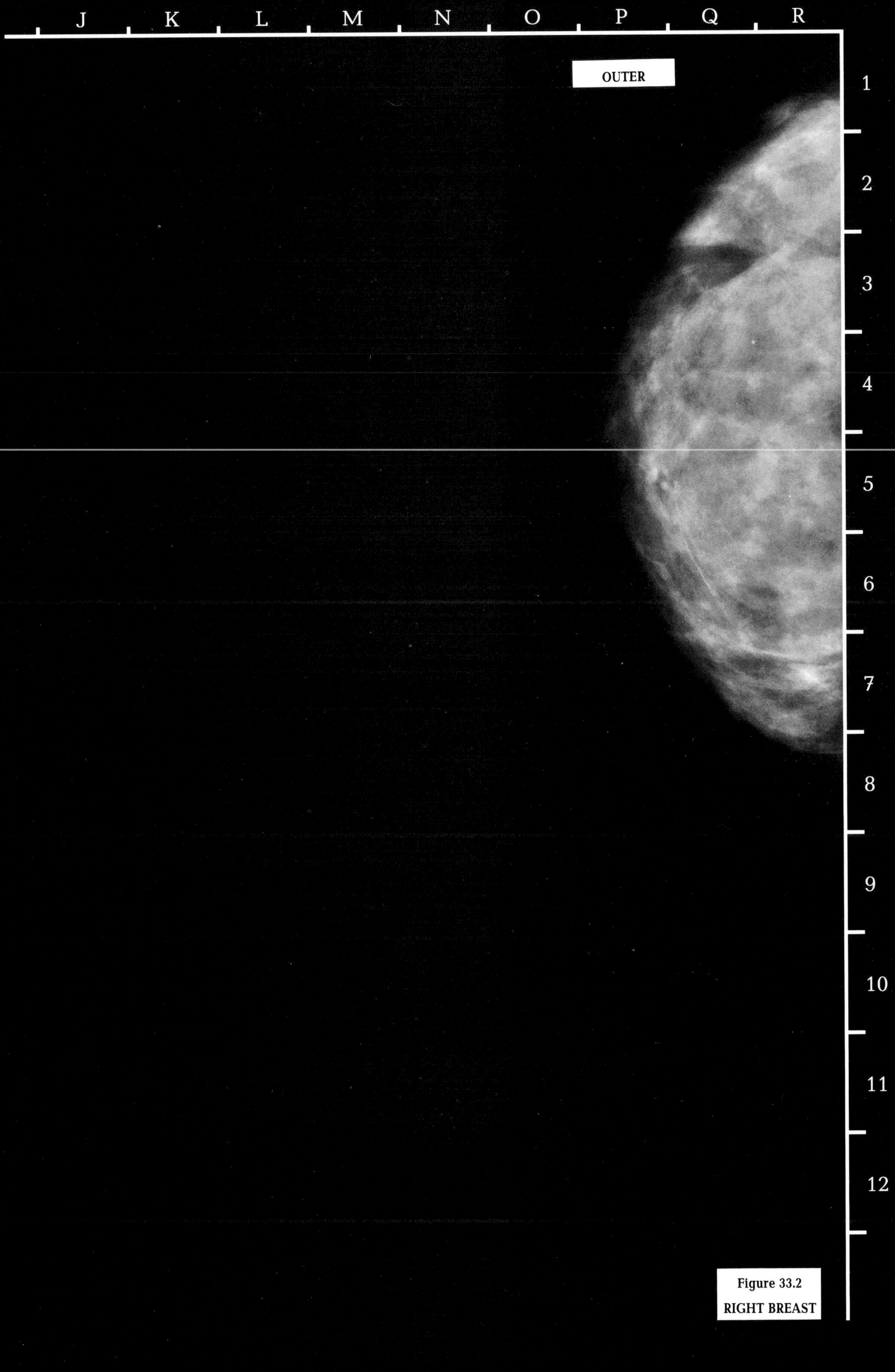

J   K   L   M   N   O   P   Q   R

OUTER

1

2

3

4

5

6

7

8

9

10

11

12

Figure 33.2
RIGHT BREAST

Findings

There is an area of architectural distortion in the upper–outer quadrant (G5), (R3).

Discussion

A cephalocaudal spot-compression view confirmed the localized, spiculated architectural distortion in the outer hemisphere *(Figure 33.3)*. The lesion was localized with a hookwire and removed. The histologic specimens showed varied manifestations of fibrocystic changes with fibrosis *(Figure 33.4)*.

Fibrocystic changes comprise a group of proliferative disorders of the breast related to hormonal stimulation, and include fibrosis, cysts, epithelial hyperplasia, papillomatosis and apocrine metaplasia. The most commonly affected age group is 35–50 years. Epidemiologists have been concerned that fibrocystic changes may carry an increased risk of breast carcinoma. However, recent investigations indicate that women who have had breast biopsies that disclose nonproliferative fibrocystic changes are not at increased risk for subsequent development of carcinoma.[36] This group of disorders includes cysts and apocrine changes. Approximately 25 percent of biopsied women with fibrocystic changes have hyperplastic lesions without atypia, and for these women the risk is 1.5–2 times that of the general population. Only about 4 percent of women have hyperplastic lesions with atypia, and for these women the relative risk of subsequent carcinoma is 4–5 times that of the general population.[108] Since almost all premenopausal women have fibrocystic changes, most of which are not associated with an increased risk of breast cancer, the term 'fibrocystic disease' should be replaced by 'fibrocystic changes'. Moreover, since these terms are histologic in origin, they should not be used in mammography; rather, the appearance should be merely described ('dense and nodular parenchyma').[68]

When there is a prominent fibrotic element the fibrocystic process undergoes retraction, resulting in architectural distortion as seen in this case. Microcalcifications may also occur as a result of an active secretory process. Some clinical features that favor fibrocystic changes over carcinoma include bilateral involvement, multiple nodules, symptoms of pain and tenderness prior to the menstrual period, generally younger age, and regression during pregnancy.

Mammographically, fibrocystic changes may mimic carcinoma when a fibrotic retractive process causes architectural distortion, or when microcalcifications or a mass is present. In many cases, carcinoma cannot be excluded with certainty, and a biopsy must be performed.

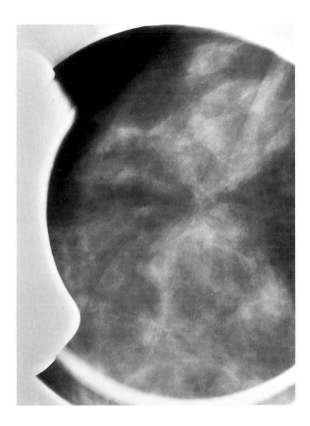

Figure 33.3

Cephalocaudal spot-compression view. The architectural distortion is due to radiating spicules. No mass is evident.

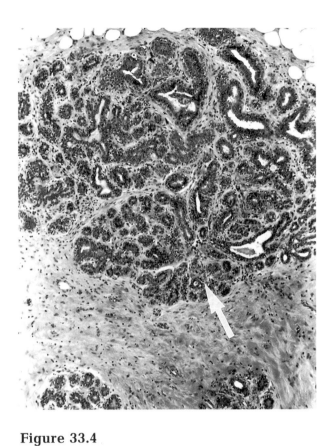

Figure 33.4

Low-power histologic specimen. This section shows early phase of adenosis with enlarged hyperplastic lobule (arrow). The fibrosis is assumed to be responsible for the retraction of the parenchyma seen in the mammogram. **Diagnosis**: Sclerosing adenosis.

Case 34

This 70-year-old woman was asymptomatic.

Films: Right *(Figure 34.1)* and left *(Figure 34.2)* mediolateral mammograms.

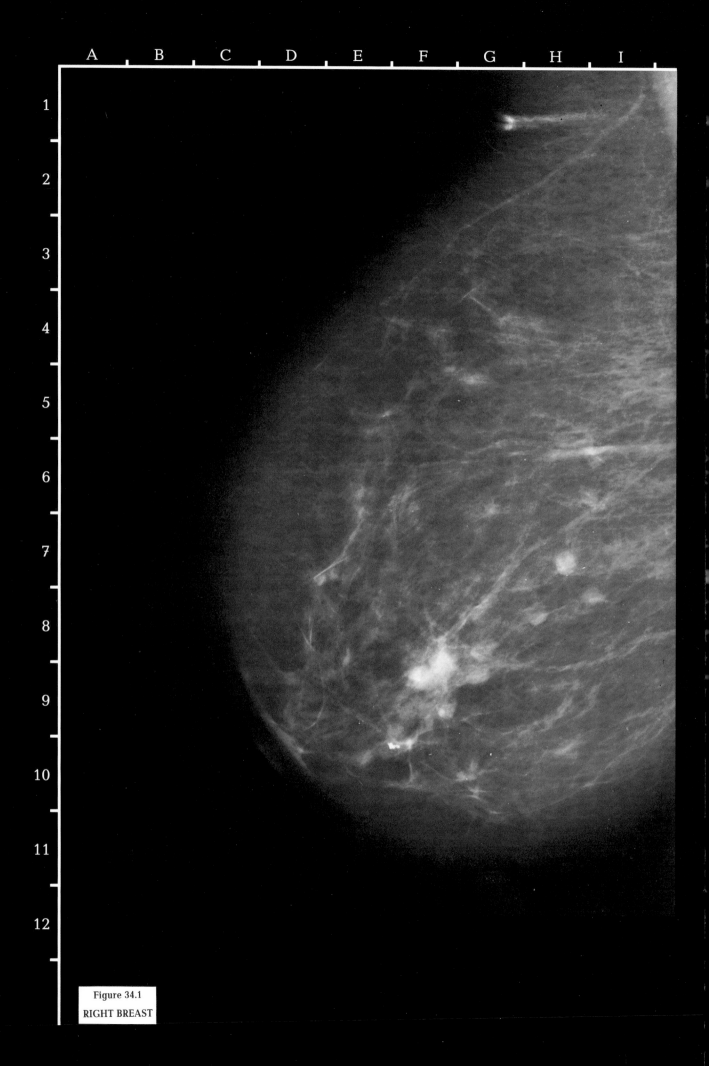

Figure 34.1
RIGHT BREAST

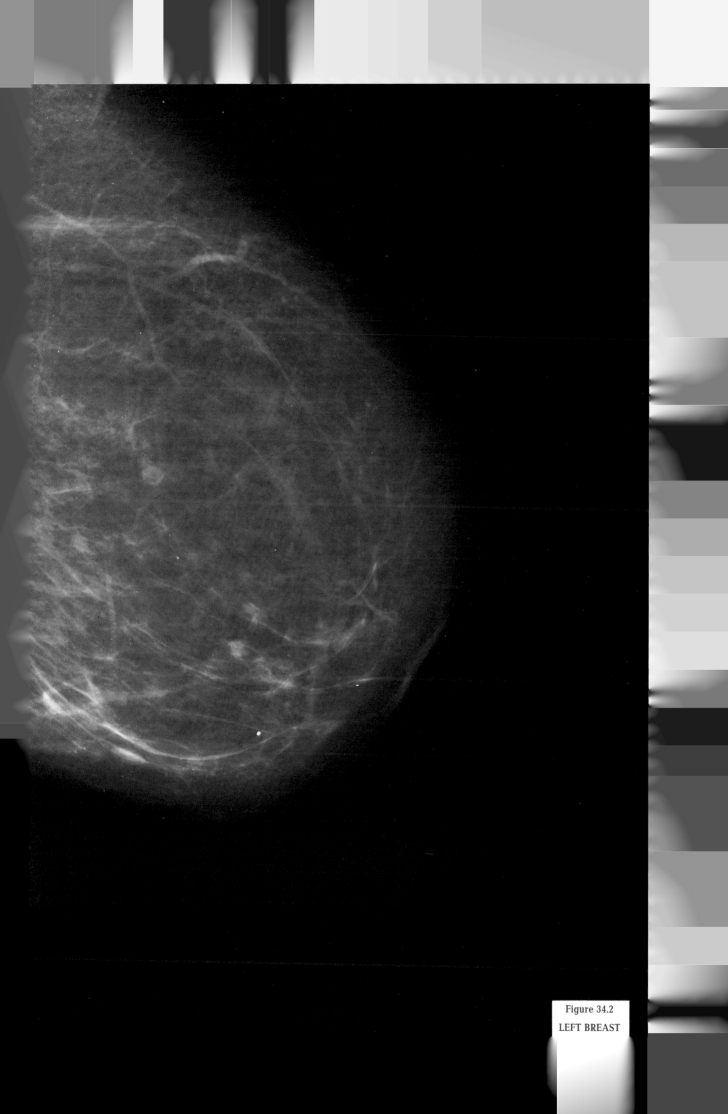

Figure 34.2
LEFT BREAST

Findings

There are benign-appearing densities throughout both breasts. An area of asymmetric increased density and architectural distortion is present in the right breast (F9). There is also a benign secretory calcification in the right breast (F10).

Discussion

The well-defined densities were felt to be benign, possibly fibroadenomas, cysts or papillomas. Cysts would be unusual in a woman aged 70, unless she was on hormone-replacement therapy. The asymmetric density in the right breast was identified in

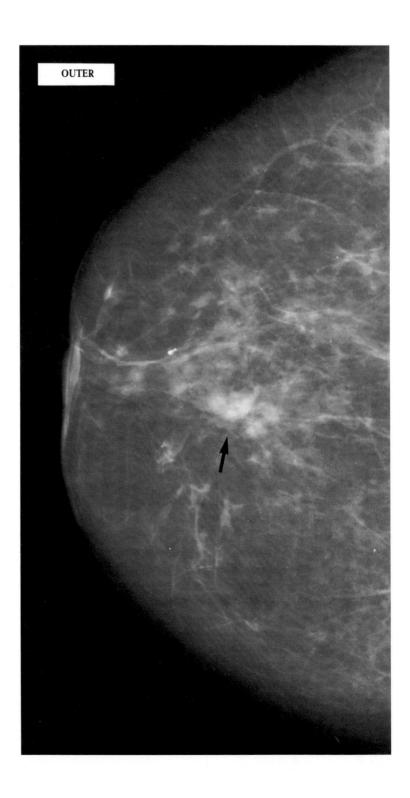

Figure 34.3

Cephalocaudal view of right breast confirms the presence of an asymmetric density (arrow) and architectural distortion.

the cephalocaudal mammogram *(Figures 34.3 and 34.4)*. Biopsy was recommended. The pathologic diagnosis was infiltrating ductal carcinoma *(Figure 34.5)*. Several of the small, well-circumscribed nodules were included in the surgical specimen, and on histologic examination proved to represent ductal papillomatosis *(Figure 34.6)*.

Papillomatosis and intraductal papillomas are common breast lesions that differ in some respects.[54] Lying within the spectrum of fibrocystic changes, papillomatosis is a benign condition found within the duct system. Papillomatosis or epitheliosis refers to epithelial proliferation of the small ducts and ductules. The epithelial cells vary

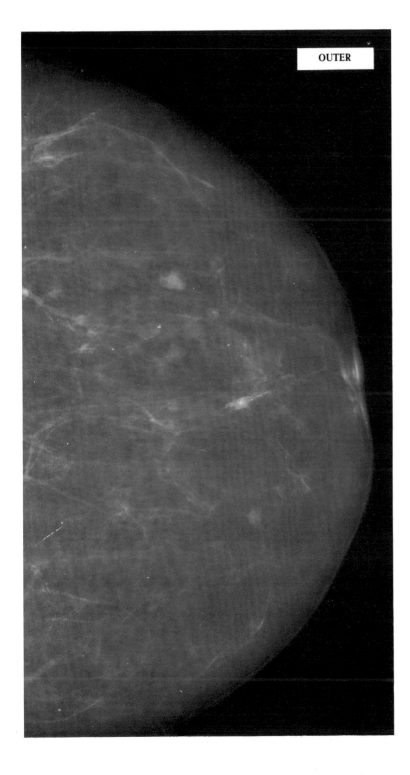

OUTER

Figure 34.4

Cephalocaudal view of left breast for comparison.

from papillary projections to cribriform patterns or solid sheets. They are not supported by fibrovascular stalks. Intraductal papillomas, on the other hand, occur in large ducts and are supported by fibrovascular cores which sometimes undergo fibrosis and hyalinization, and may result in a pseudoinvasive histologic pattern. Papillomatosis without atypia is not associated with an increased risk of carcinoma. Mammographically, papillomatosis tends to be distributed throughout the parenchyma of both breasts and may be associated with fine calcifications.[31] Solitary papillomas tend to occur in the subareolar region and are the most common cause of a bloody discharge. Solitary papillomas are not believed to be premalignant.[91] However, multiple intraductal papillomas have been identified as a separate condition that may carry an increased risk for the development of breast carcinoma.[54]

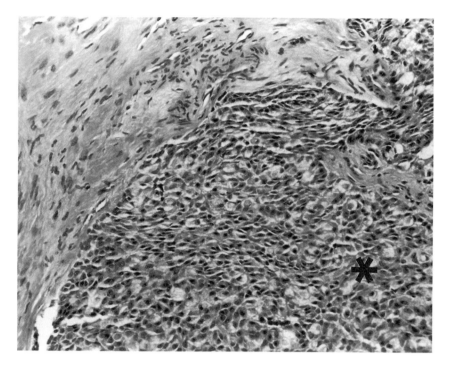

Figure 34.5

Low-power histologic section of carcinoma. There is extensive infiltration by sheets of malignant cells (asterisk) extending into the surrounding stroma. **Diagnosis**: Infiltrating ductal carcinoma.

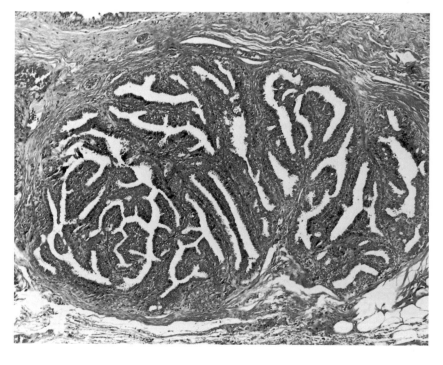

Figure 34.6

Low-power histologic section of intraductal papilloma. The lining epithelium supported by fibrovascular stalks is thrown into papillary projections within the lumen of the duct. The duct is distended but intact. The result is a smooth nodular density in the mammogram. **Diagnosis**: Intraductal papilloma.

Case 35

This 56-year-old woman with bilateral silicone implants had undergone left tylectomy (lumpectomy) and radiotherapy for carcinoma 2 years ago. She complained of a lump at the site of the previous tylectomy.

Films: Right *(Figure 35.1)* and left *(Figure 35.2)* mediolateral oblique mammograms.

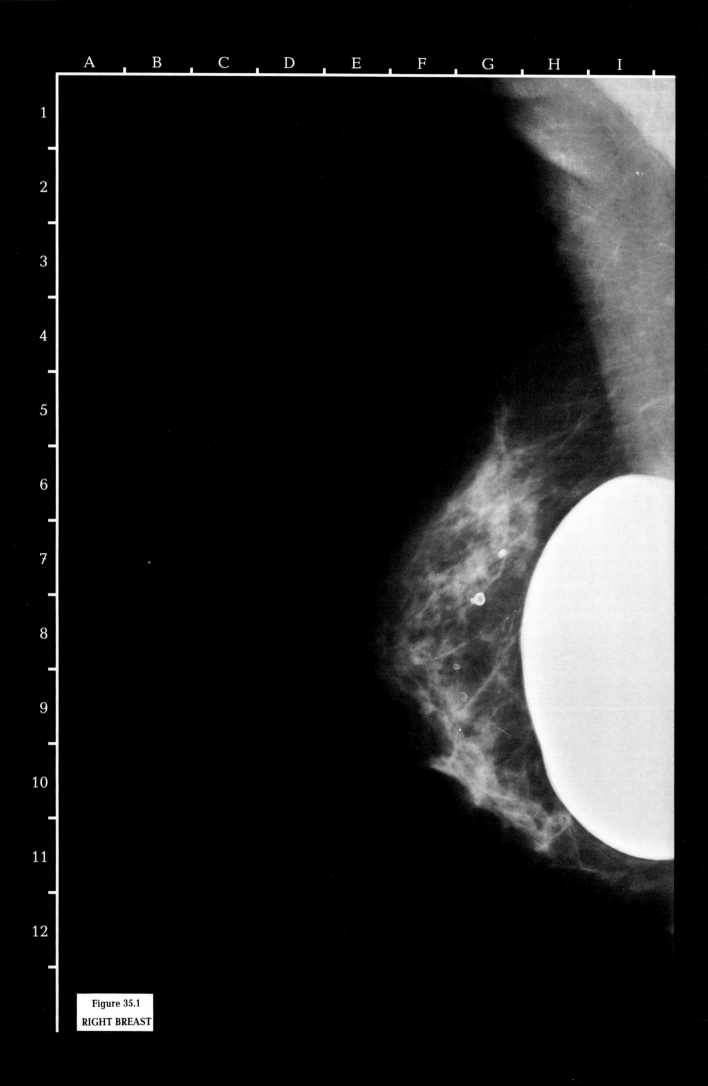

Figure 35.1
RIGHT BREAST

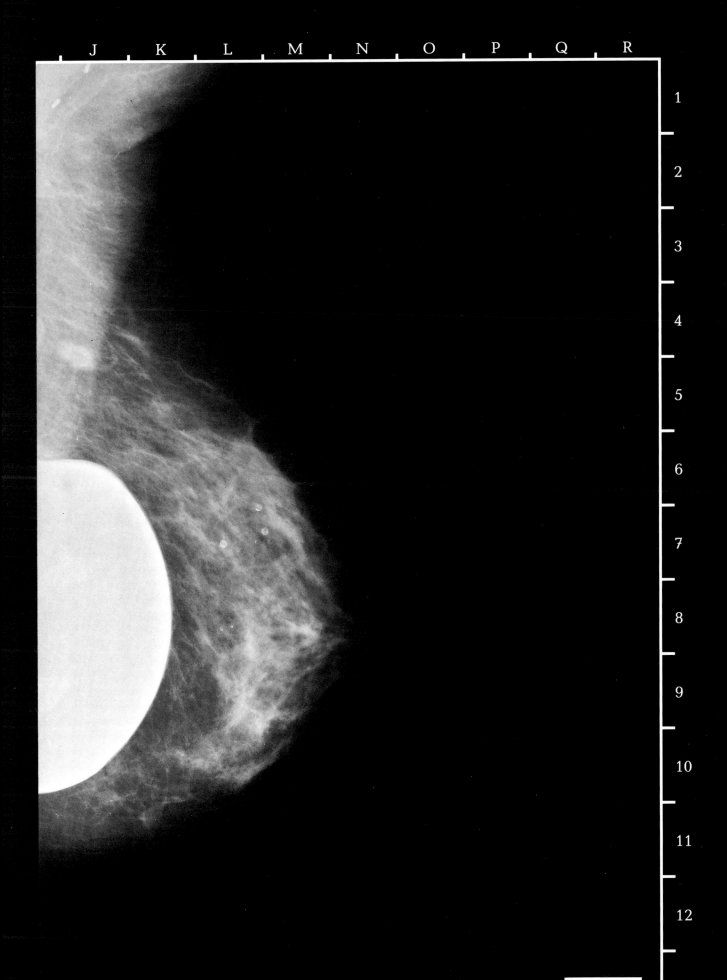

J K L M N O P Q R

1
2
3
4
5
6
7
8
9
10
11
12

Figure 35.2
LEFT BREAST

Findings

Bilateral benign coarse calcifications contain lucent centers. There are two moderately well circumscribed densities (J4), one of which is only partially visualized at the posterior edge of the film, in the upper hemisphere of the left breast.

Discussion

The ill-defined densities *(Figure 35.3)* were at the site of the palpable abnormality. Biopsy revealed that both densities were composed of colloid carcinoma *(Figure 35.4)*.

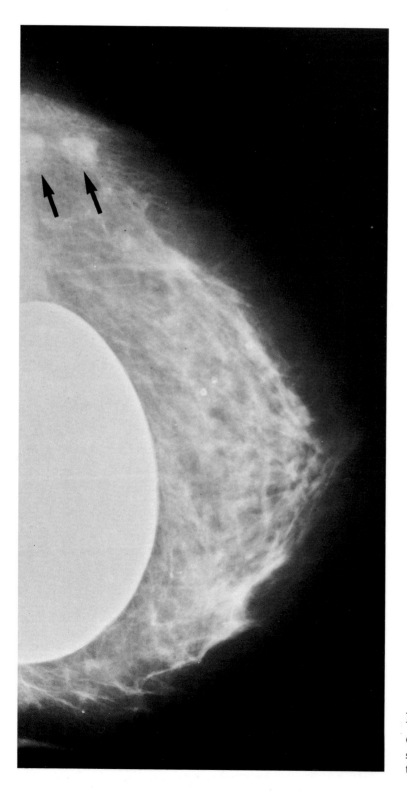

Figure 35.3

Close-up, mediolateral mammogram. The suspicious densities (arrows) are close to the chest wall.

Silicone implants do not place a woman at a higher risk than normal for breast cancer, but they may be associated with the development of several complications.[30] In addition, silicone implants, because of their density, may obscure overlying breast tissue and compromise the accuracy of the mammographic examination.[32] The usefulness of mammography in patients with augmentation mammoplasty depends on the size of the implants (larger implants obscuring more of the breast tissue and, after preventing optimal breast compression, making mammography less useful), and the quality of parenchyma (patients with a larger volume of parenchyma are more likely to benefit from mammography than those with a small volume). It is important that the referring physician is aware of the limitations of mammography in patients with implants. Recent improvements in mammography and positioning have made the imaging of implants more effective.[40]

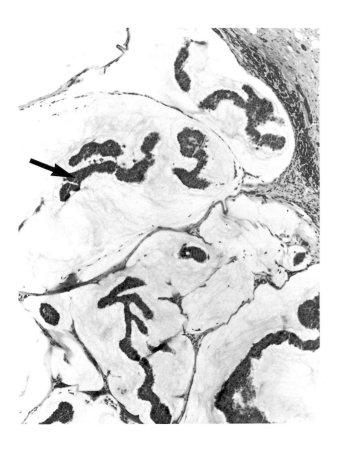

Figure 35.4

Low-power histologic section. There are nests of malignant epithelial cells (arrow) within large pools of mucin. **Diagnosis**: Mucinous (colloid) carcinoma.

Case 36

This 40-year-old woman had a lump in the lower–outer quadrant of the left breast.

Films: Right *(Figure 36.1)* and left *(Figure 36.2)* mediolateral mammograms.

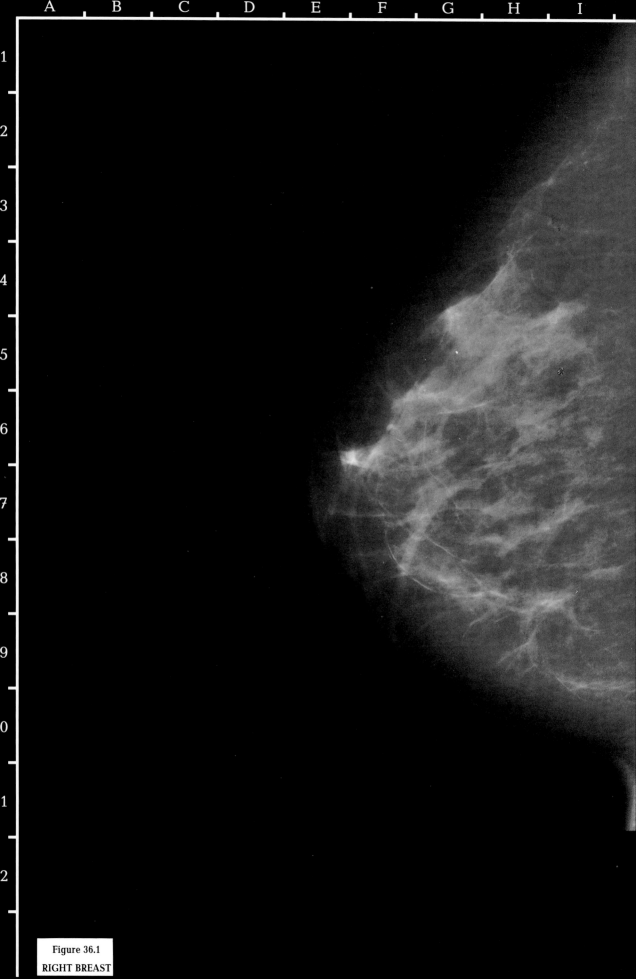

Figure 36.1
RIGHT BREAST

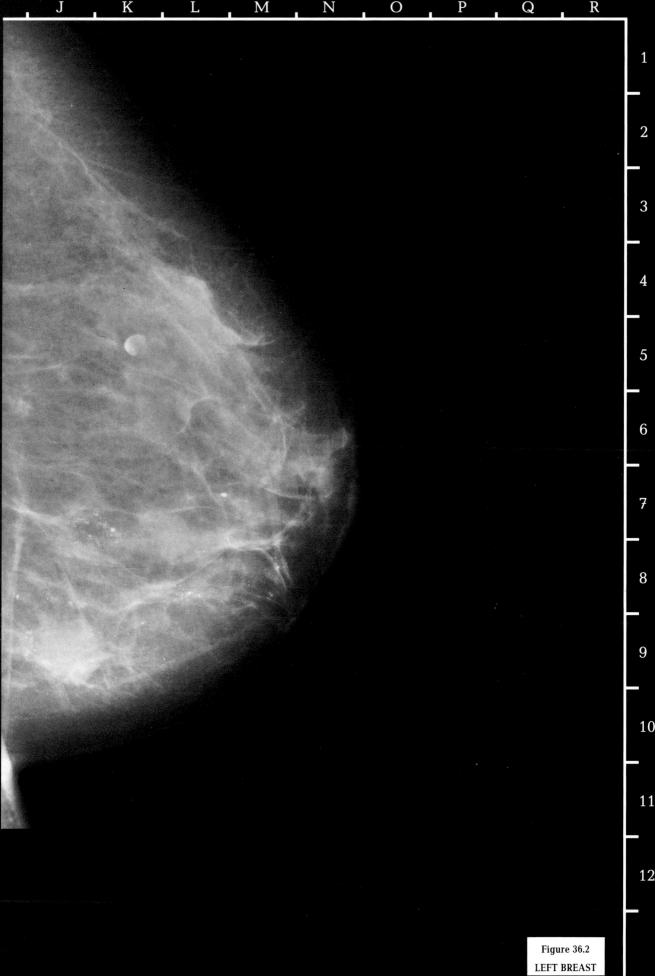

Figure 36.2
LEFT BREAST

Findings

In the left breast, there is a 1.5 cm dense mass (J9) with ill-defined margins in the lower hemisphere. In addition, there are several foci of clustered microcalcifications (J7), (J9), (L8), (M8). A benign coarse calcification is present in the upper hemisphere (K5).

Discussion

The irregular 1.5 cm mass in the left breast is at the site of the palpable lump. Its ill-defined posterior margin makes it suspicious for malignancy. The clustered microcalcifications are also suspicious for carcinoma. The prebiopsy mammographic diagnosis was multifocal carcinoma ('multifocal' meaning that 2 cm or more of normal tissue separated foci of tumor). Biopsy confirmed multifocal infiltrating ductal carcinoma.

The case illustrates the importance of performance of a mammogram before biopsy of a palpable lump.[50,112] The pretreatment mammogram is more precise than physical examination in the depiction of the size and extent of the tumor, and the presence of multifocal lesions. In this case, the mammogram showed that the tumor extended beyond the area of the palpable mass. All tumor foci should be removed if breast-conserving surgery is to be successful.[110] If the extent of the tumor is widespread or multicentric (widely separated tumor foci involving more than one quadrant of the breast), the patient may be considered suitable for breast conservation because of the

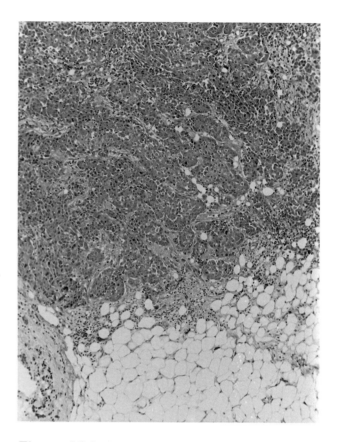

Figure 36.3

There are sheets and clusters of malignant epithelial cells infiltrating the fat and fibrous stroma. **Diagnosis**: Infiltrating ductal carcinoma.

likelihood of excessive deformity. Tylectomy (lumpectomy) was not possible in this case due to the extent of the tumor, and a modified radical mastectomy was performed.

Case 37

This 39-year-old woman complained of pain in both breasts.

Films: Right *(Figure 37.1)* and left *(Figure 37.2)* mediolateral oblique and right *(Figure 37.3)* and left *(Figure 37.4)* cephalocaudal mammograms.

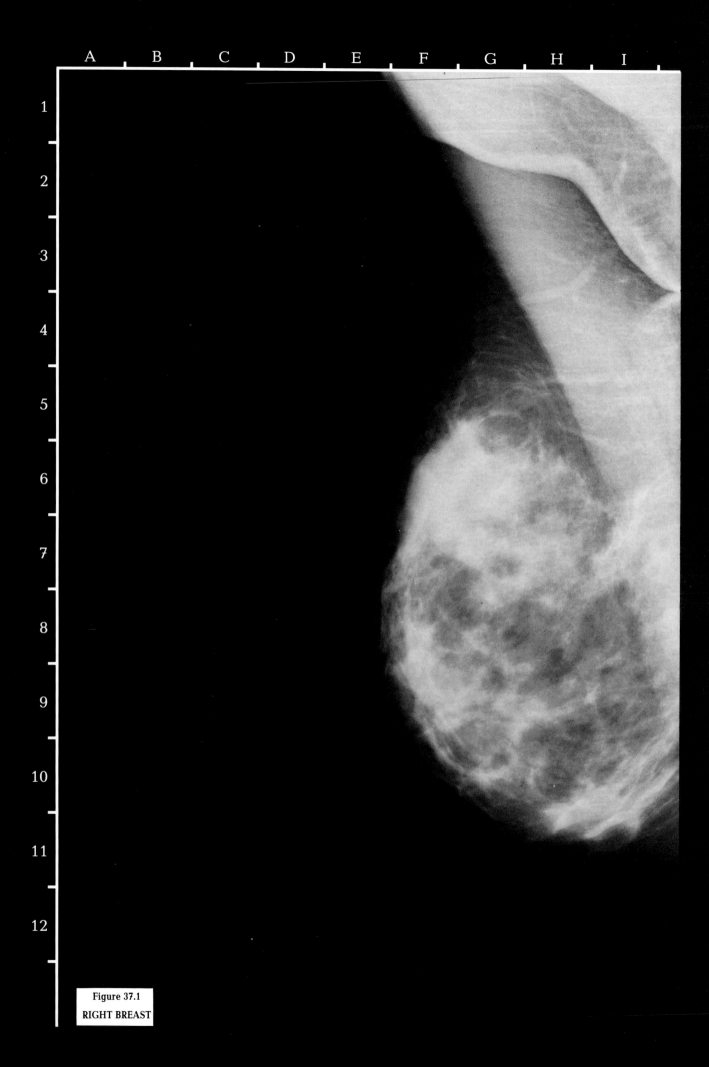

Figure 37.1
RIGHT BREAST

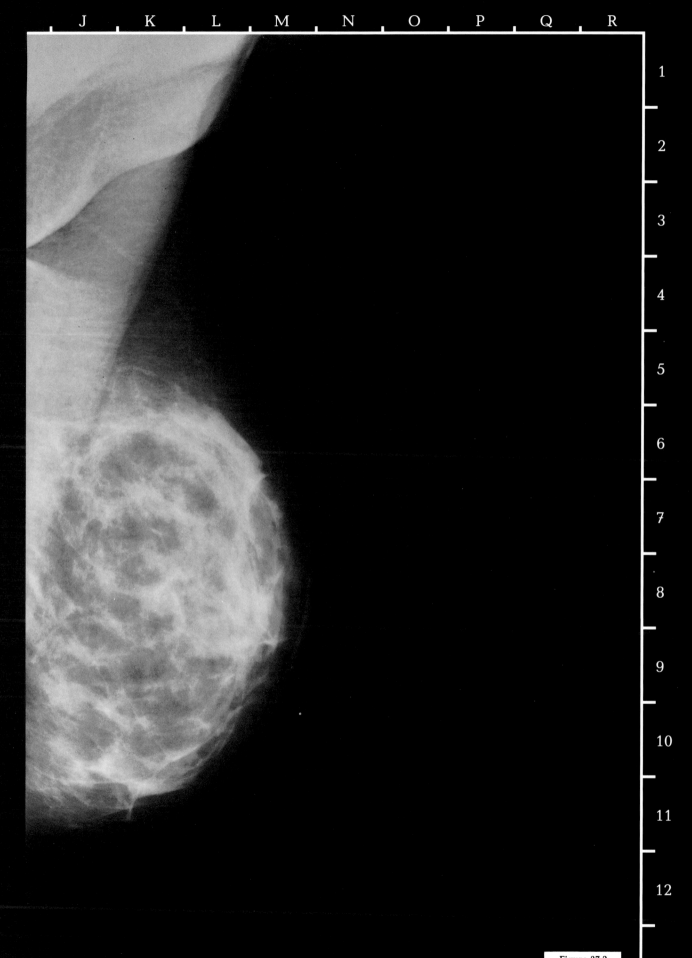

Figure 37.2
LEFT BREAST

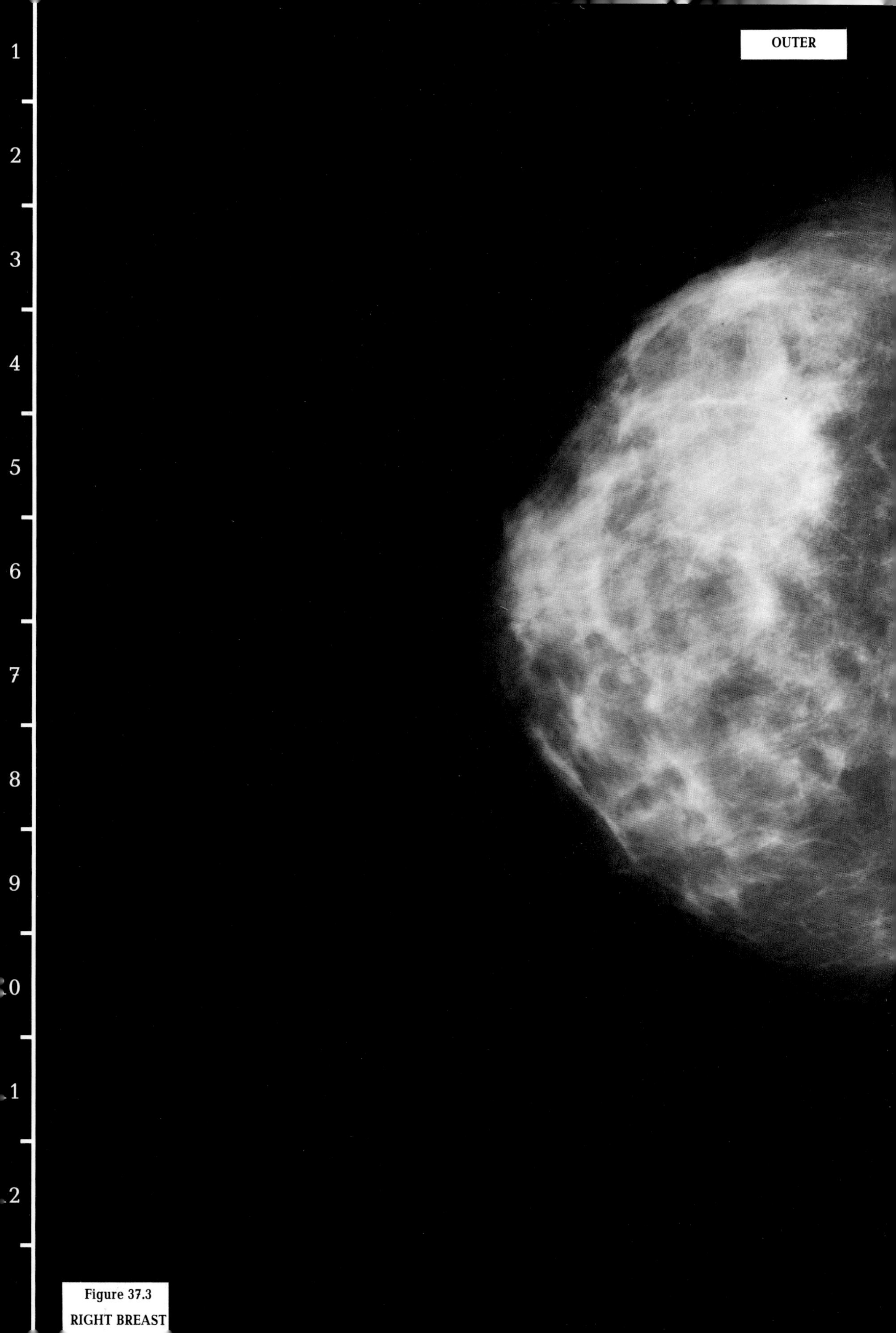

1

2

3

4

5

6

7

8

9

0

1

2

Figure 37.3
RIGHT BREAST

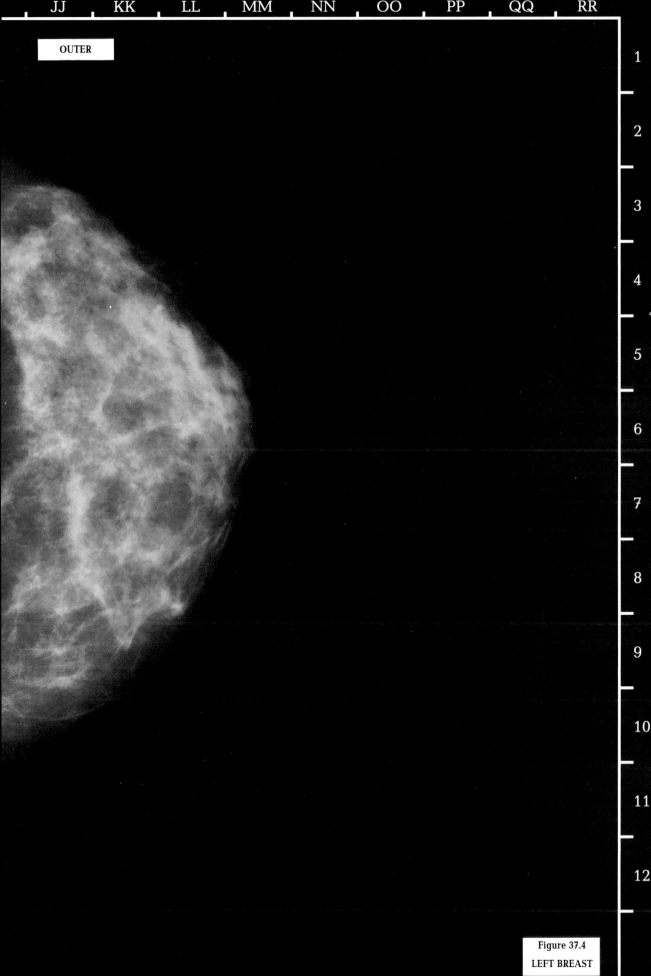

JJ   KK   LL   MM   NN   OO   PP   QQ   RR

OUTER

1
2
3
4
5
6
7
8
9
10
11
12

Figure 37.4
LEFT BREAST

Findings

There is an asymmetric focus of increased parenchymal density in the upper–outer quadrant of the right breast (G6), (HH5).

Discussion

A focus of asymmetric parenchymal density may result from superimposition of normal parenchymal tissue in any one mammographic view, and therefore must be seen in two views to be considered of possible significance. Because breasts may normally show some asymmetry, to be considered suspicious for malignancy an asymmetric density should be associated with architectural distortion, microcalcifications or a palpable abnormality.[79] In this mammogram, there was architectural distortion at the periphery of the asymmetric density, and the distortion persisted in spot-compression films. Biopsy revealed infiltrating ductal carcinoma.

Case 38

This 44-year-old woman was referred for a mammographic abnormality in her right breast.

Films: Right mediolateral *(Figure 38.1)* and cephalocaudal *(Figure 38.2)* mammograms.

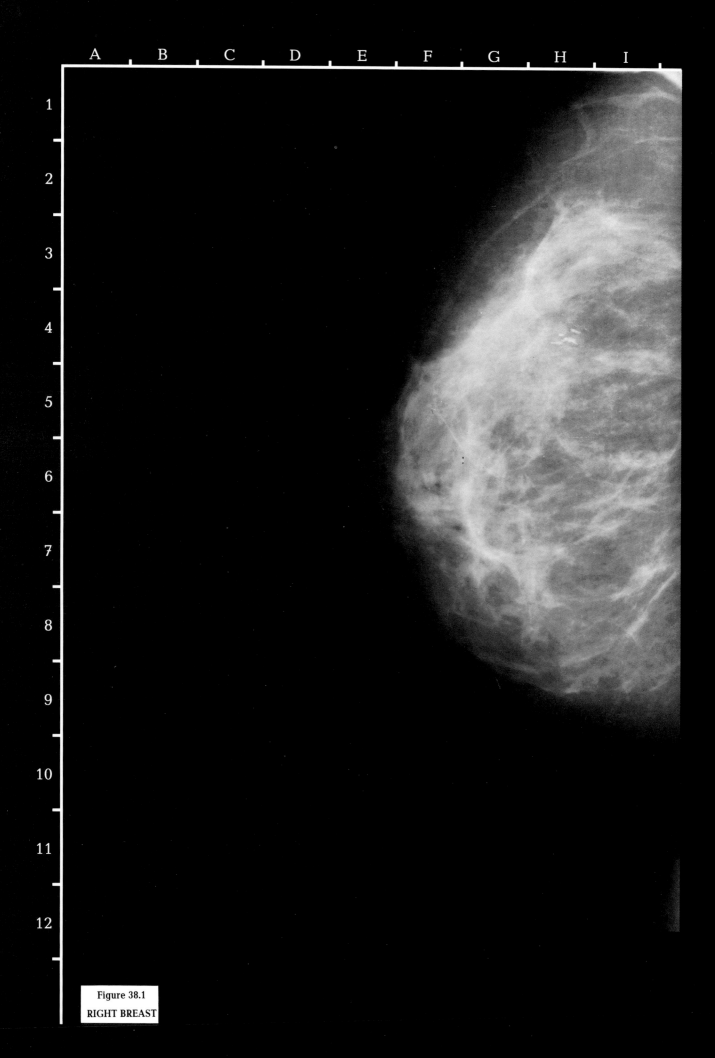

Figure 38.1
RIGHT BREAST

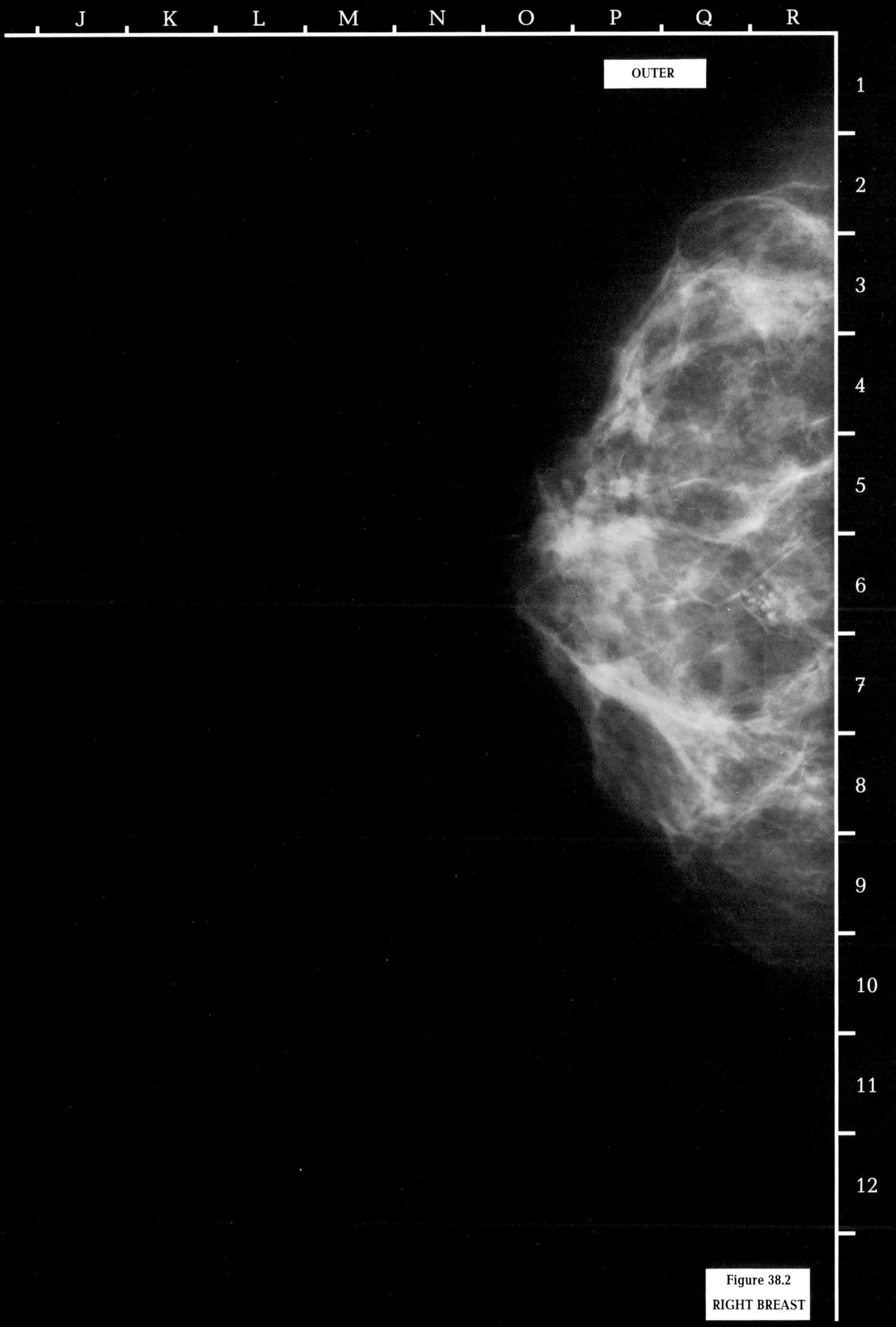

J K L M N O P Q R

OUTER

1
2
3
4
5
6
7
8
9
10
11
12

Figure 38.2
RIGHT BREAST

Findings

A group of calcifications is identified on both mediolateral (H4) and cephalocaudal (R6) views.

Discussion

The calcifications change their configuration from mediolateral to cephalocaudal views. In the mediolateral view *(Figure 38.1)* they are well defined, linear or curvilinear, while in the cephalocaudal view *(Figure 38.2)* they are round, low-density 'smudges'. These are the characteristic features of gravity-dependent sedimented calcium, or milk of calcium within microcysts.[82,130] Because they behave in a fashion similar to the sediment at the bottom of a cup of tea, they are referred to as 'teacup' calcifications.

Sedimented calcium in the breast is a benign condition that occurs in 4–6 percent of women undergoing mammography. The calcifications are usually bilateral, and may occur in scattered or locally clustered fashion.[66] True mediolateral (horizontal beam) mammograms may be necessary to definitively characterize the calcifications as benign. Fine-detail magnification views, obtained in both true mediolateral and cephalocaudal projections, are helpful in making the diagnosis.[87]

Case 39

This 70-year-old woman had a lump in the right breast.

Films: Right *(Figure 39.1)* and left *(Figure 39.2)* lateral mammograms.

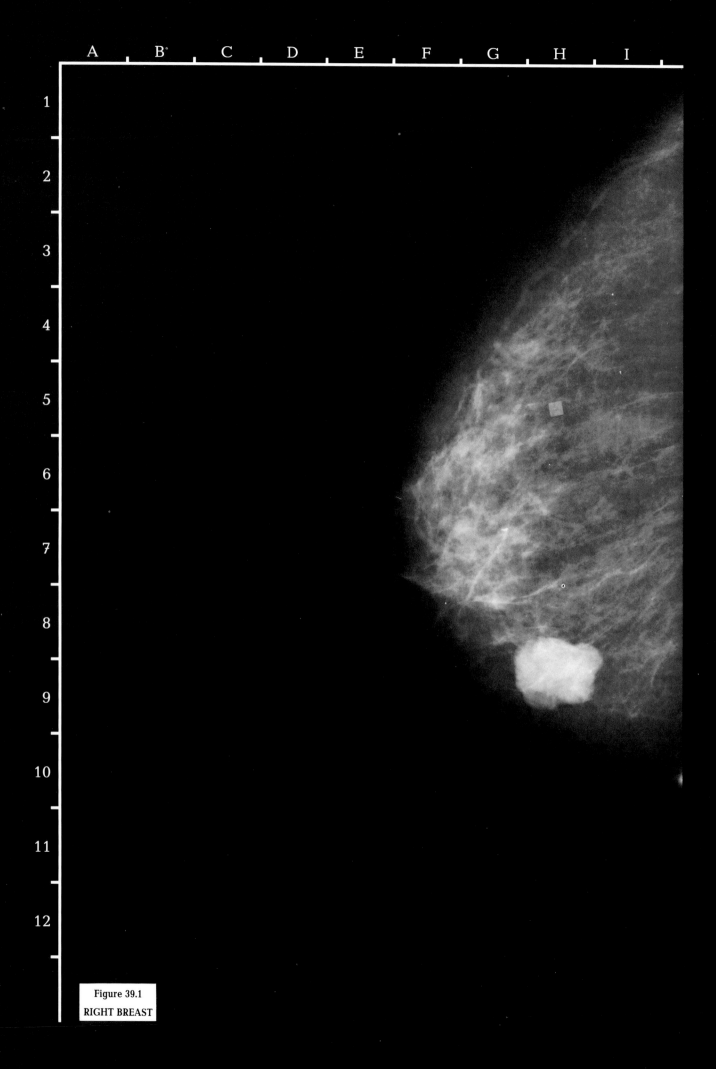

Figure 39.1
RIGHT BREAST

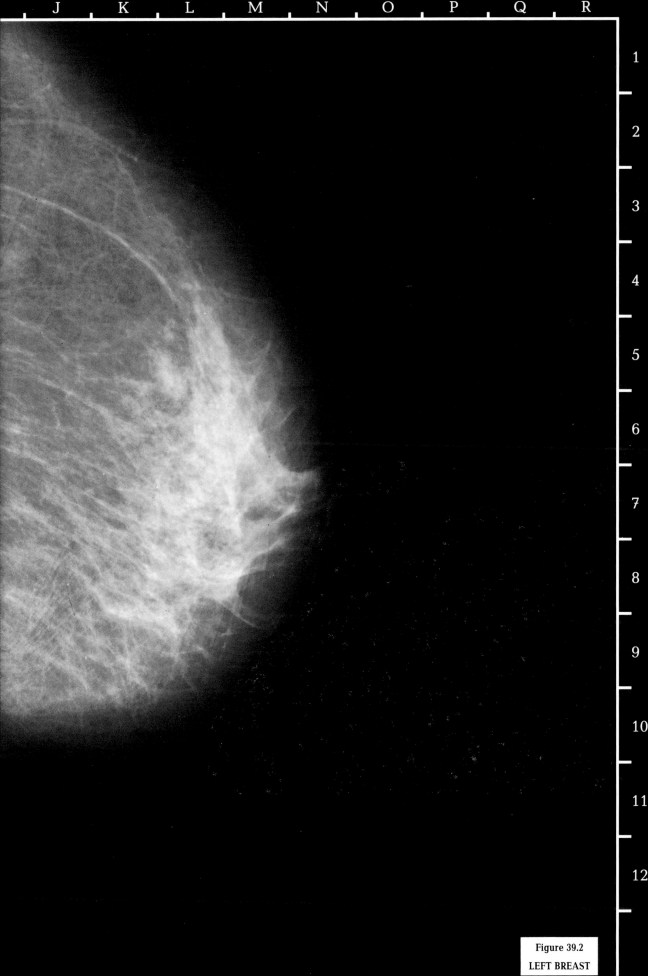

J   K   L   M   N   O   P   Q   R

1
2
3
4
5
6
7
8
9
10
11
12

Figure 39.2
LEFT BREAST

Findings

A 2 cm mass (H9) is seen in the lower hemisphere of the right breast. The mass is lobulated and has smooth margins. In addition, there is a benign-appearing solitary calcification (G7) and a 3 mm radiolucent square object (H5).

The left breast was unremarkable.

Discussion

In a younger woman, the lobulated, well-circumscribed mass would most probably be a fibroadenoma. However, in an older woman, well-circumscribed malignant tumors such as well-circumscribed ductal carcinoma, medullary, papillary carcinoma or mucinous carcinomas must also be considered. Biopsy was recommended. The histologic diagnosis was medullary carcinoma *(Figure 39.3)*.

Medullary carcinoma makes up less than 2 percent of all breast cancers.[54] Because it is not associated with the desmoplastic reaction often associated with ductal carcinoma, on palpation it is usually softer. Medullary carcinomas grow centrifugally along a broad front, are mammographically well circumscribed, and tend to be relatively large at the time of diagnosis. The prognosis for carcinomas with a well-delimited, rounded or lobulated contour is better than for carcinomas with a grossly irregular or stellate contour showing radial projections into the periphery.[81,103,116]

The small radiolucent square is a thermoluminescent dosimeter (TLD). This dose-monitoring chip is placed on the surface of the breast prior to X-ray exposure. After exposure, the TLD is returned by mail to the monitoring laboratory, where the midbreast or average glandular dose is estimated according to the type of mammographic equipment used and the thickness of the exposed breast.

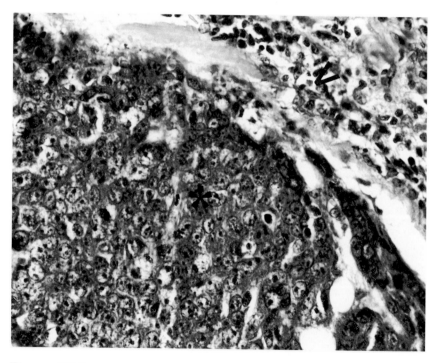

Figure 39.3

Low-power histologic section. The tumor is characterized by solid sheets of large cells (asterisk) and a moderate lymphocytic infiltrate (L). **Diagnosis**: Medullary carcinoma.

Case 40

This 35-year-old woman was referred for screening mammography.

Films: Left mediolateral oblique *(Figure 40.1)* and left cephalocaudal *(Figure 40.2)* mammograms.

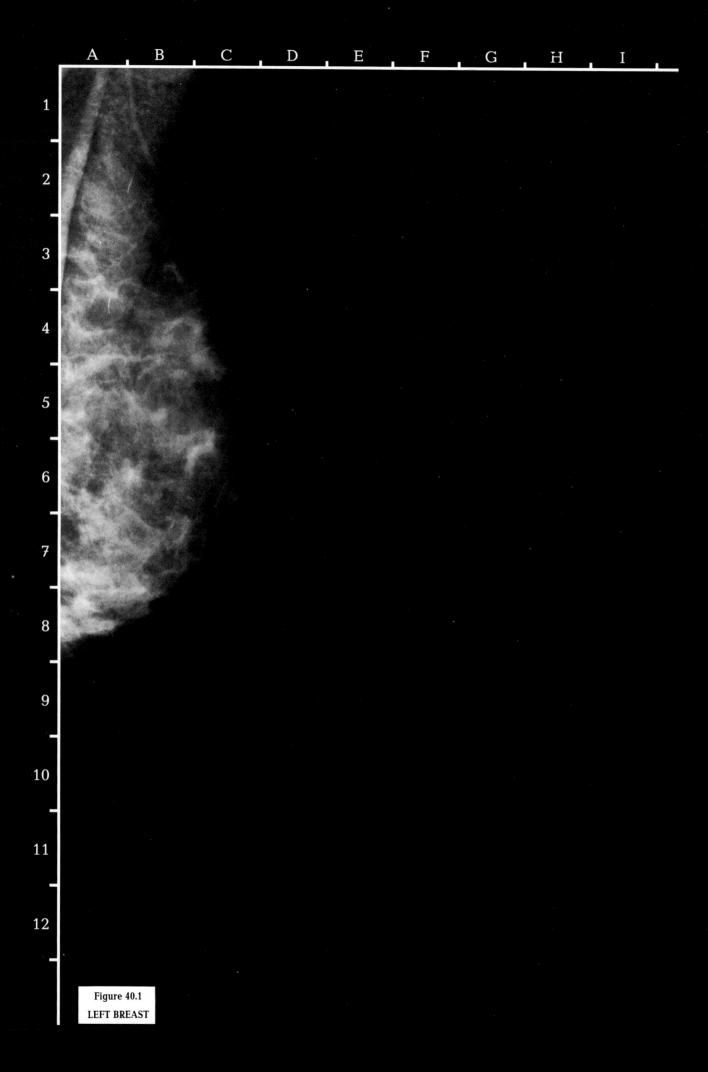

Figure 40.1
LEFT BREAST

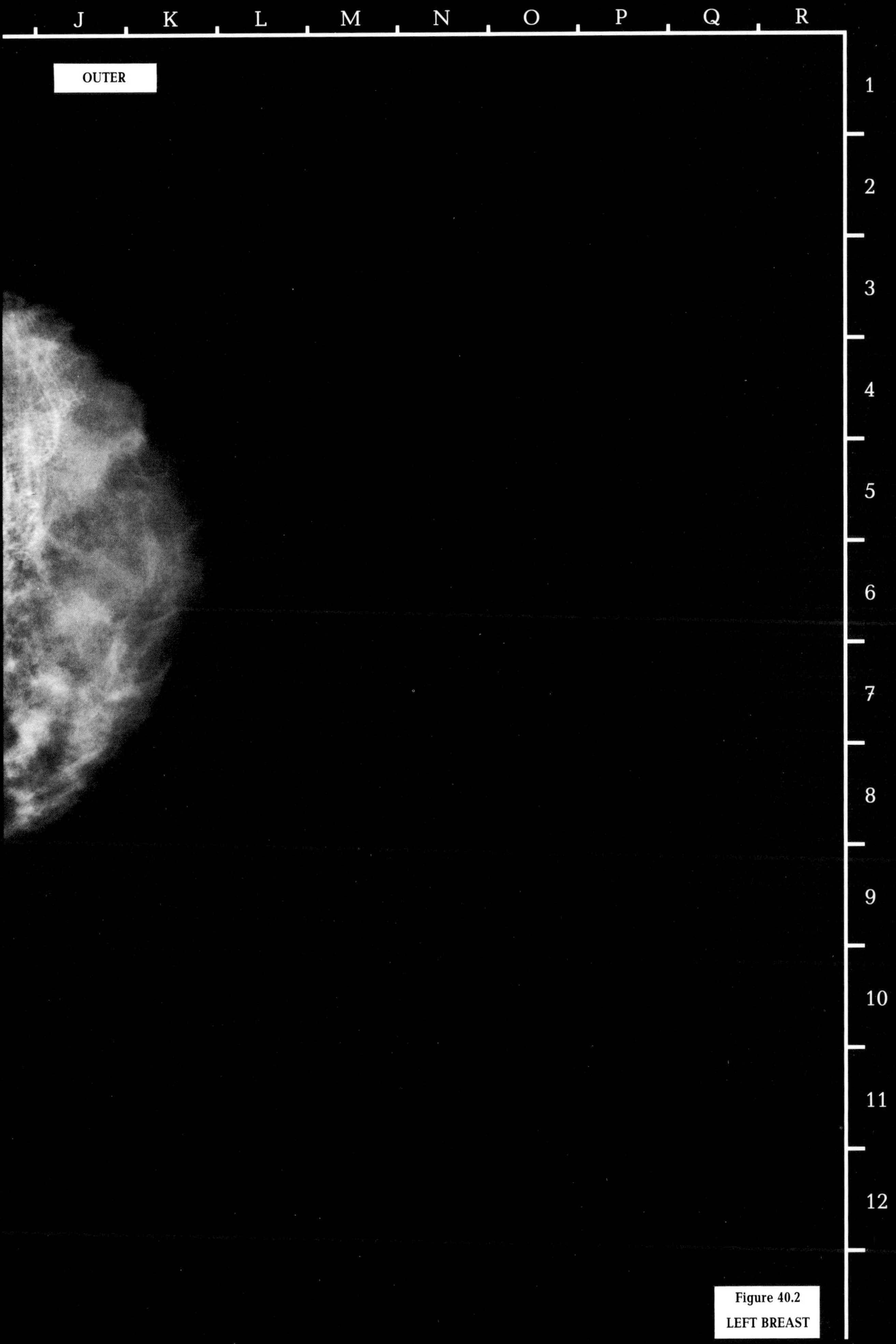

J K L M N O P Q R

OUTER

1
2
3
4
5
6
7
8
9
10
11
12

Figure 40.2
LEFT BREAST

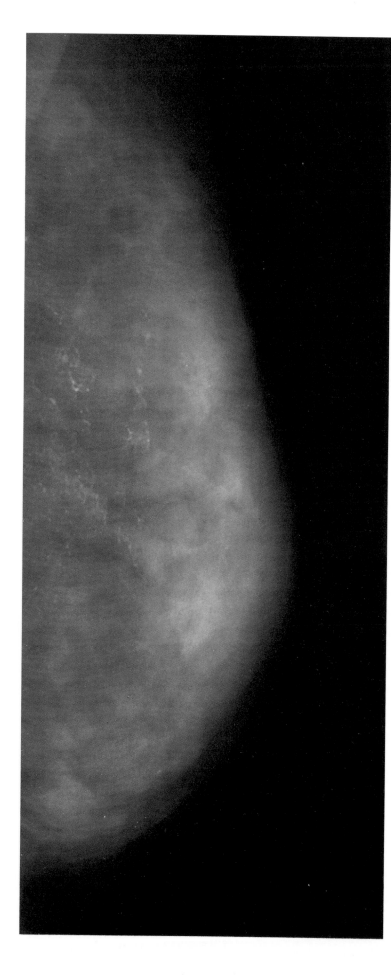

Figure 40.3

Electrocardiographic electrode lead paste on skin.

Findings

In the cephalocaudal view there appear to be numerous calcifications in the outer hemisphere of the left breast (J4). These are not seen in the oblique projection.

Discussion

The possibility of an artifact should be considered because the apparent calcifications are seen in only one view. Indeed, the patient's long hair had been superimposed on the breast at the time of the cephalocaudal exposure. With the hair away from the breast the cephalocaudal mammogram was repeated. The abnormality had disappeared.

Other artifacts that may simulate calcifications in mammograms include talc powder, zinc oxide ointment, electrocardiographic electrode paste *(Figure 40.3)*, fingerprints on intensifying screens *(Figure 40.4)* and tattoo pigments *(Figure 40.5)*.

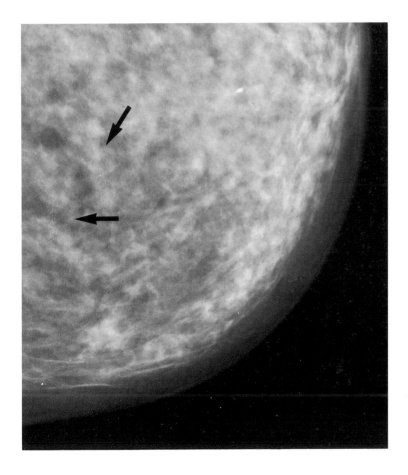

Figure 40.4

Close-up of fingerprints (arrows) on intensifying screen simulating calcifications in film.

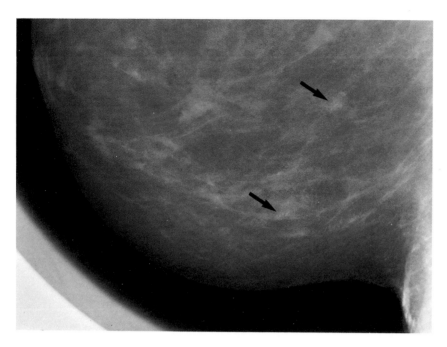

Figure 40.5

Pigment in tattoos (arrows) simulates calcifications.

Case 41

This 62-year-old woman was referred because of an abnormal screening mammogram.

Films: Right *(Figure 41.1)* and left *(Figure 41.2)* cephalocaudal mammograms.

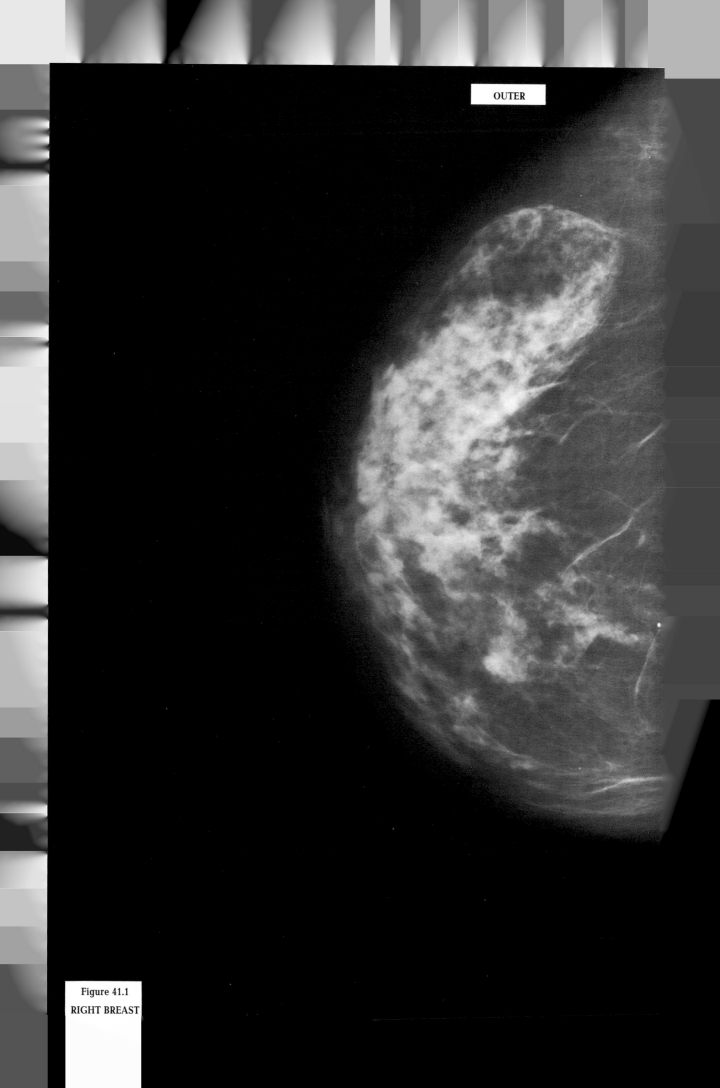

OUTER

Figure 41.1
RIGHT BREAST

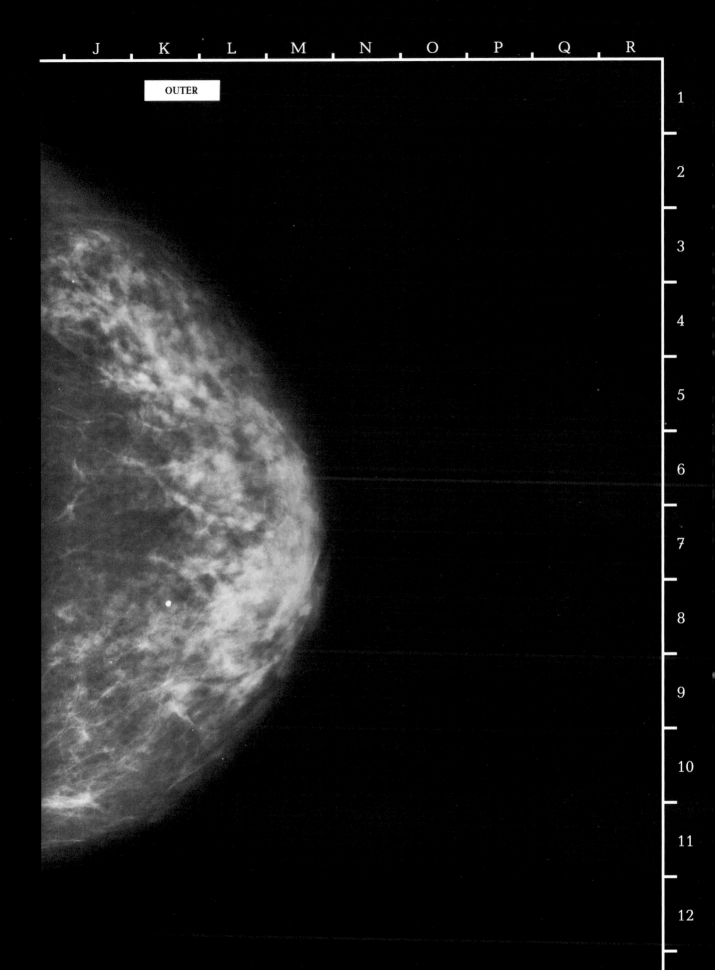

J K L M N O P Q R

OUTER

1
2
3
4
5
6
7
8
9
10
11
12

Figure 41.2
LEFT BREAST

Findings

There are small clusters of calcifications in the right breast (including H5 and H8) and in the left breast (including J9).

Discussion

Biopsies had been recommended for each of the clusters of calcification. However, clusters in the right breast could not be localized in a lateral view *(Figure 41.3)*, while the most suspicious cluster in the left breast could be identified in a lateral view *(Figure 41.4)*. A fine-detail magnified lateral view of the right breast disclosed the two suspicious clusters and verified that they had features suspicious for malignancy *(Figure 41.5)*. The pathologic diagnosis was multiple foci of lobular carcinoma in situ (LCIS) *(Figures 41.6 and 41.7)*.

LCIS is a proliferation in the acini and/or terminal ductules. It is also called 'lobular neoplasia', which is a less alarming term than carcinoma in situ, and it leaves more flexibility for treatment.[124,125] It occurs predominantly in premenopausal women, and the lobular component can regress to some degree after menopause. It has a great propensity to multicentricity and bilaterality. Because the involved lobules and ductules are small and widely dispersed, LCIS rarely forms a palpable tumor and is difficult to detect clinically. It does not metastasize, but it does predispose to the development of invasive carcinoma. In a longitudinal survey of 99 patients with LCIS treated by local excision and followed over 24 years, 36.9 percent developed invasive carcinoma in the same or contralateral breast.[119] The carcinomas that developed were either ductal or lobular. The mammographic manifestations of LCIS vary, but the most common seems to be round calcifications of the lobular type.[138] The origin of these calcifications is uncertain, but may be due to extension of LCIS into ductules leading to their obstruction, with resultant inspissation and calcification of the secretions from adjacent normal lobules.[148]

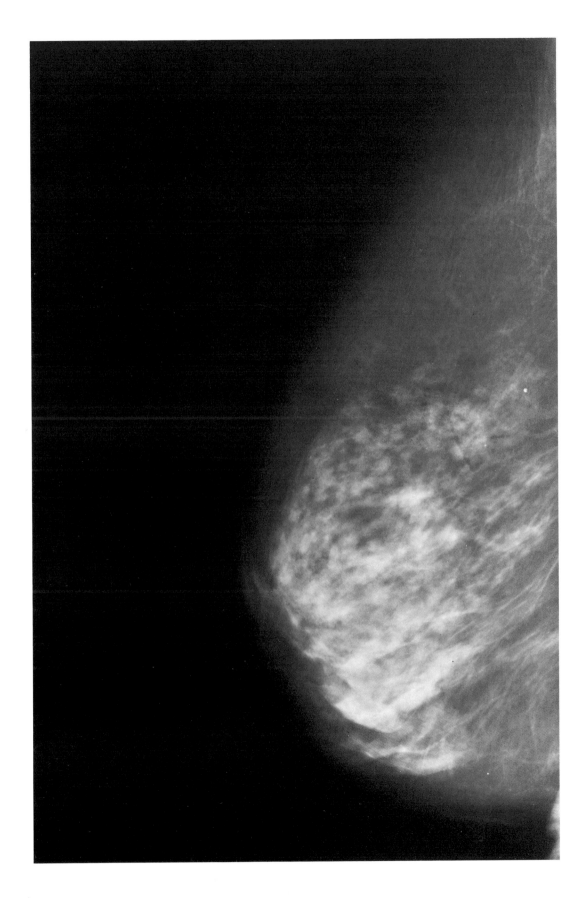

Figure 41.3

Lateral view of right breast. The calcifications are not identified.

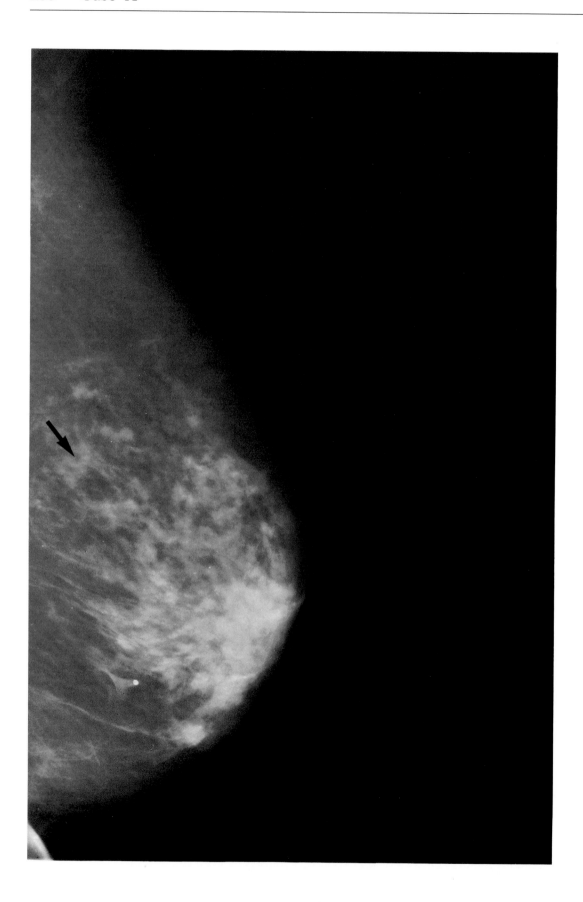

Figure 41.4

Lateral view of left breast. The cluster of calcifications (arrow) is in the upper hemisphere.

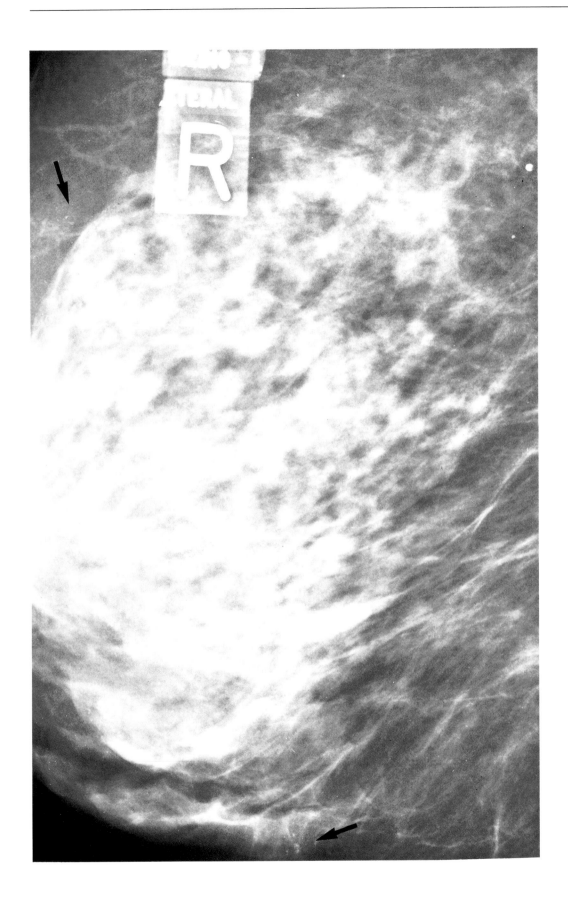

Figure 41.5

Magnification view of right breast. One cluster of calcifications is located in the upper hemisphere (arrow) and one in the lower hemisphere (arrow).

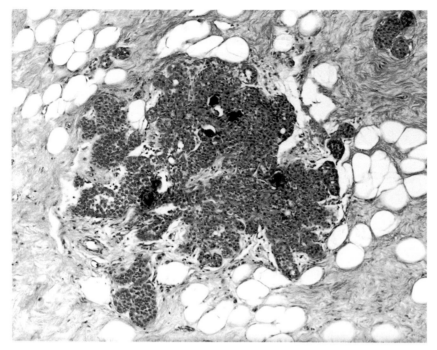

Figure 41.6

Low-power histologic section. Neoplastic cells fill the lumens of the acini and form solid, rounded units. **Diagnosis**: Lobular carcinoma in situ.

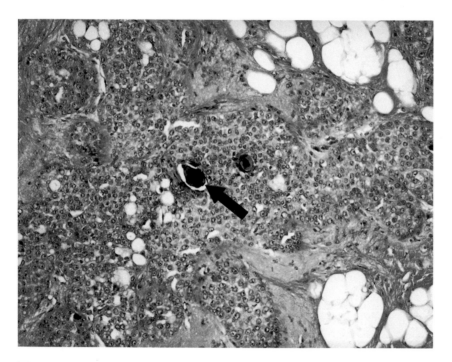

Figure 41.7

High-power histologic section. There is calcification (arrow) within the acini.

Case 42

This 59-year-old woman was referred for screening mammography.

Films: Right *(Figure 42.1)* and left *(Figure 42.2)* mediolateral oblique mammograms.

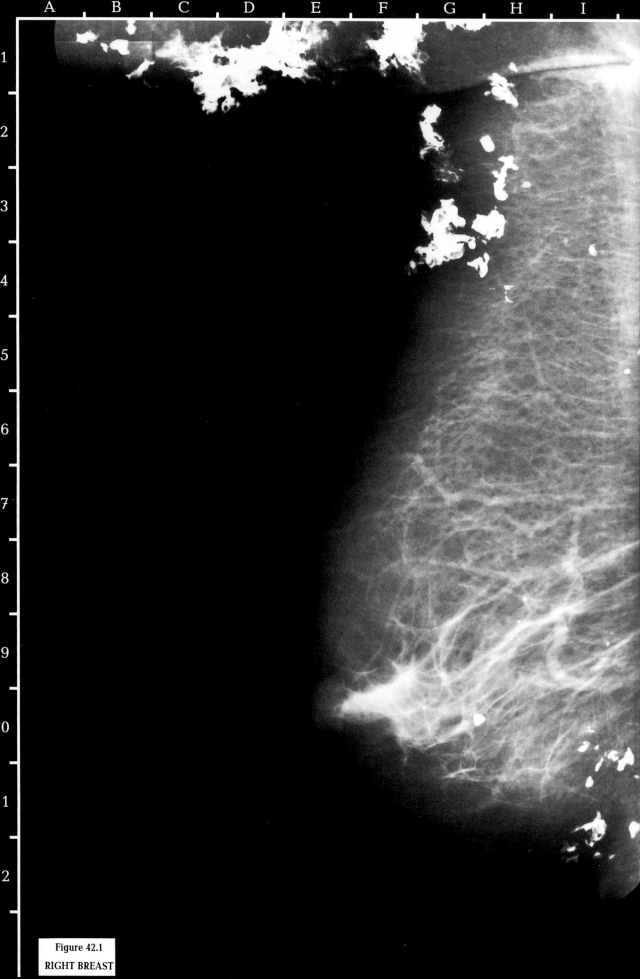

Figure 42.1
RIGHT BREAST

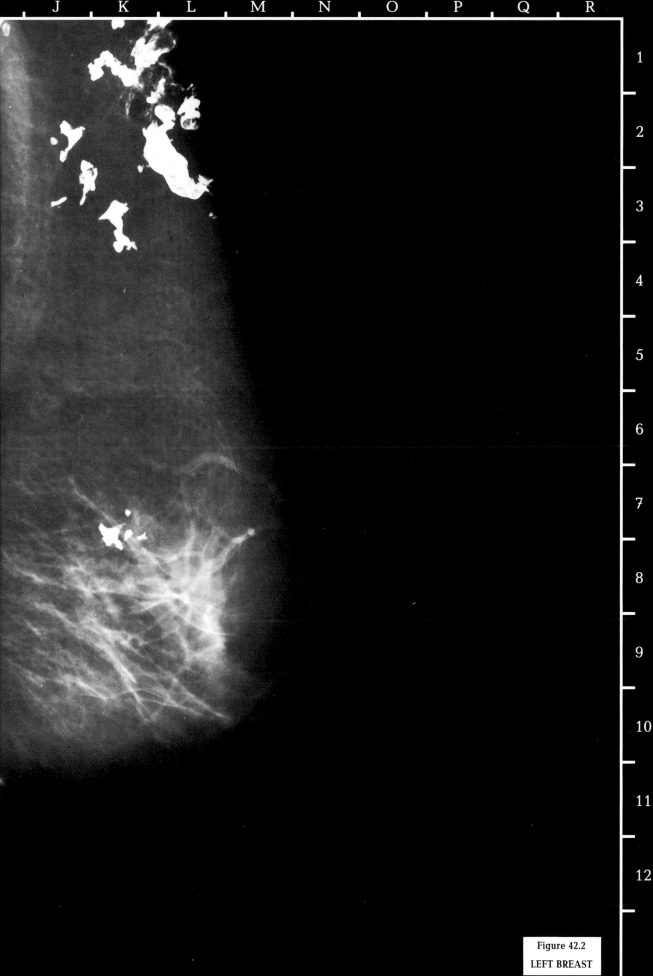

Figure 42.2
LEFT BREAST

Findings

There are coarse calcifications overlying both axillae and breasts.

Discussion

The calcifications have benign radiographic features in that they are large and dense. The patient had a history of dermatomyositis, a chronic inflammatory myopathy of uncertain origin, character-ized by degeneration of individual groups of muscle fibers with prominent interstitial infiltrates of chronic inflammatory cells.[23] It is often accompanied by a prominent skin rash which typically occurs in the malar eminences and bridge of the nose in a butterfly distribution, similar to that seen in systemic lupus erythematosus. A similar eruption may occur on the neck, forehead, shoulder, and front and back of the upper chest. With time, atrophy and fibrosis of the skin and subcutaneous tissues lead to dystrophic calcifications in the dermis, which may be shown in the mammogram, as in this case.

Case 43

This 29-year-old woman was referred for a palpable mass in the lower right breast.

Films: Right *(Figure 43.1)* and left *(Figure 43.2)* mediolateral mammograms.

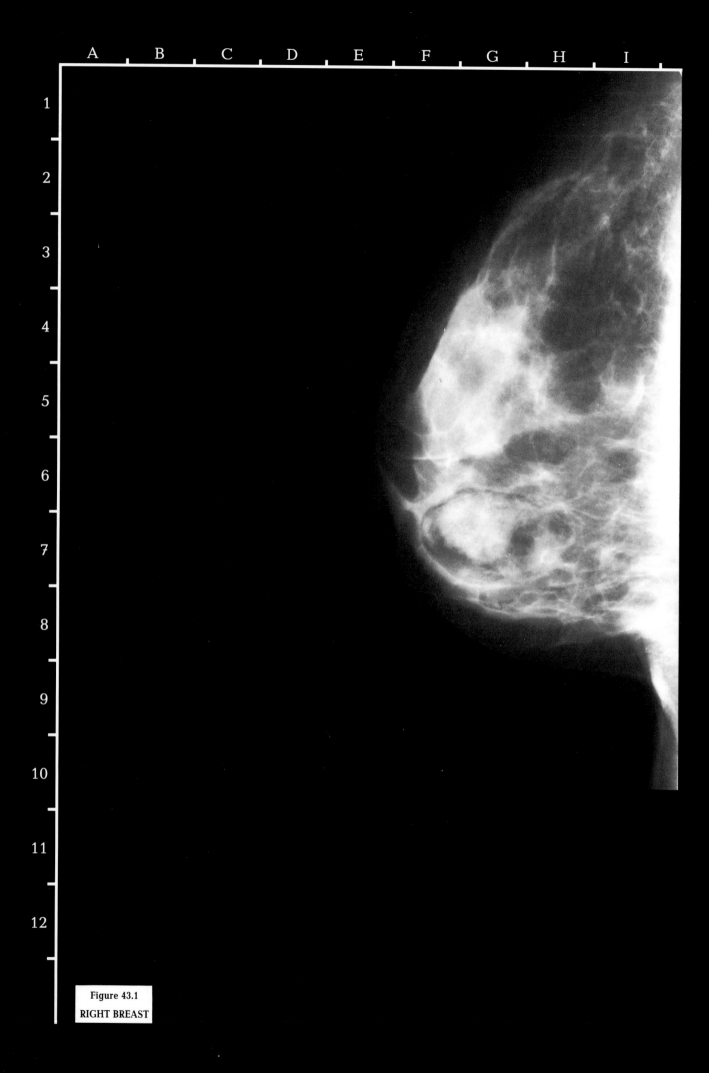

Figure 43.1
RIGHT BREAST

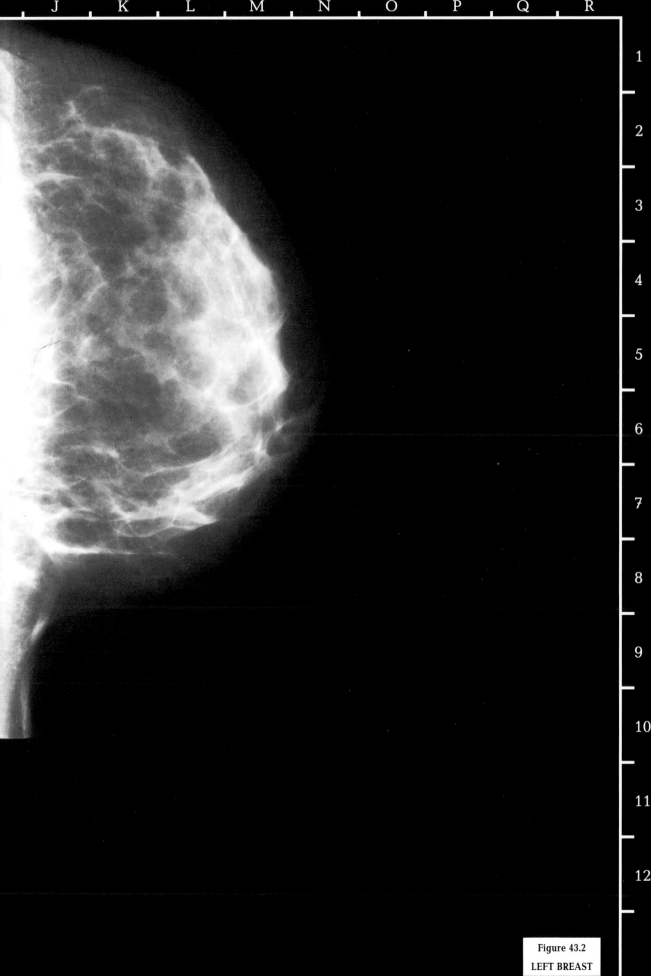

Figure 43.2
LEFT BREAST

Findings

There is a mass of mixed soft tissue and fat density in the lower hemisphere of the right breast (G7).

Discussion

The mass contains a combination of fatty and soft tissue densities, characteristic of lipofibroadenoma. There appears to be a dense capsule around the anterior aspect of the mass *(Figure 43.3)*. As the radiographic features are pathognomonic, a biopsy was not performed.

Lipofibroadenoma, also called 'hamartoma of the breast', is a benign lesion with no report of malignant degeneration.[28] Because the proportion of adipose to parenchymal components varies, the lesion may be relatively radiolucent or dense.[60,90] It is usually well defined by a thin fibrous capsule.

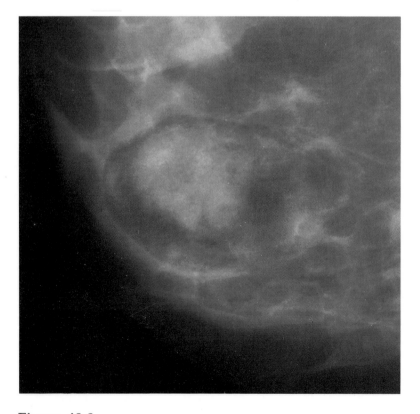

Figure 43.3

Close-up of lateral view. The lesion contains a mixture of fatty and denser tissues. A capsule is visible anteriorly.

Case 44

This 43-year-old woman was referred for two lumps in the left breast.

Films: Right *(Figure 44.1)* and left *(Figure 44.2)* mediolateral oblique mammograms.

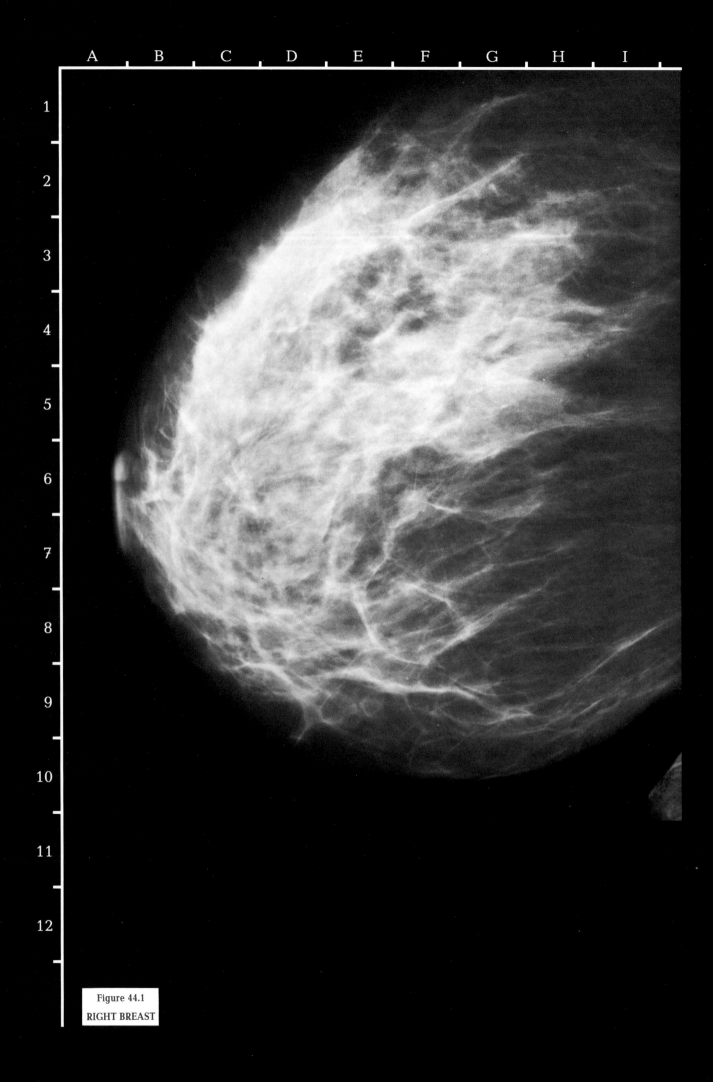

Figure 44.1
RIGHT BREAST

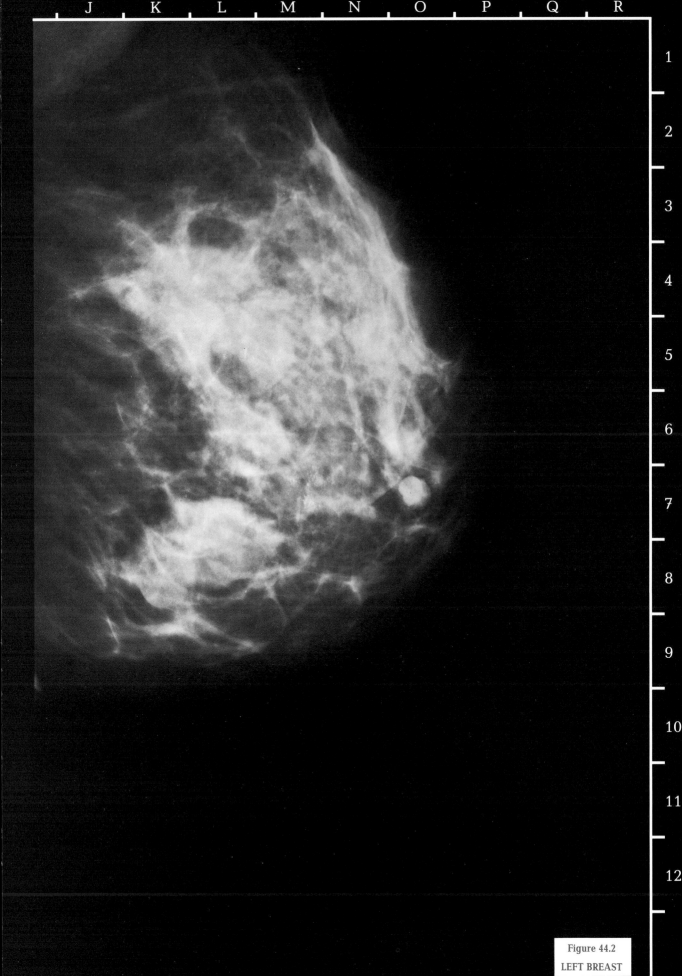

Figure 44.2
LEFT BREAST

Findings

The right breast shows two well-defined densities (D7), (F6) and three or four scattered calcifications. The left breast contains several well-defined densities (K8), (N5), (O7), two ill-defined densities (L4), (L7) and clustered calcifications (M7).

Discussion

Clinical examination was important in this case. Moles on the skin of both breasts were imaged in the mammograms as well-defined densities (Figure 44.3). The ill-defined densities on the left breast matched the sites of the palpable masses, and sonography showed that they were solid (Figure 44.4). The clustered calcifications were numerous and manifested irregular sizes and shapes, features suspicious for malignancy.

Biopsy revealed that both of the palpable masses and the clustered calcifications in the left breast represented infiltrating carcinoma. The diagnosis was multicentric carcinoma, since malignancies were found in more than one quadrant. Because the tumor was so extensive, a breast-conserving therapeutic procedure was contraindicated and a mastectomy was performed.

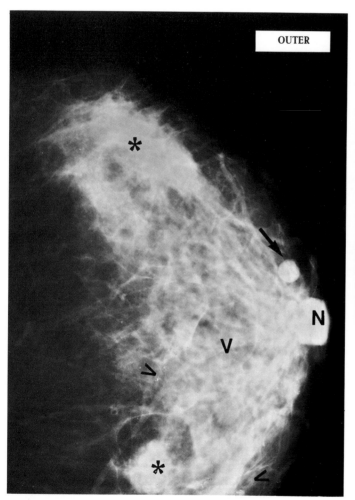

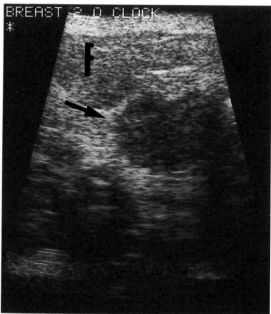

Figure 44.4

Sonography. The palpable mass (arrow) was solid, and more sonolucent than the subcutaneous fat (F).

Figure 44.3

Cephalocaudal mammogram. The two palpable masses (asterisk) are ill defined. A mole (arrow) on the surface of the breast is well defined, being surrounded by air. The nipple (N), superimposed on the image of the breast, is also surrounded by air. The clustered calcifications (open arrowheads) cover a wide area.

Case 45

This 40-year-old woman was referred for a palpable mass in her left breast.

Films: Right *(Figure 45.1)* and left *(Figure 45.2)* mediolateral mammograms.

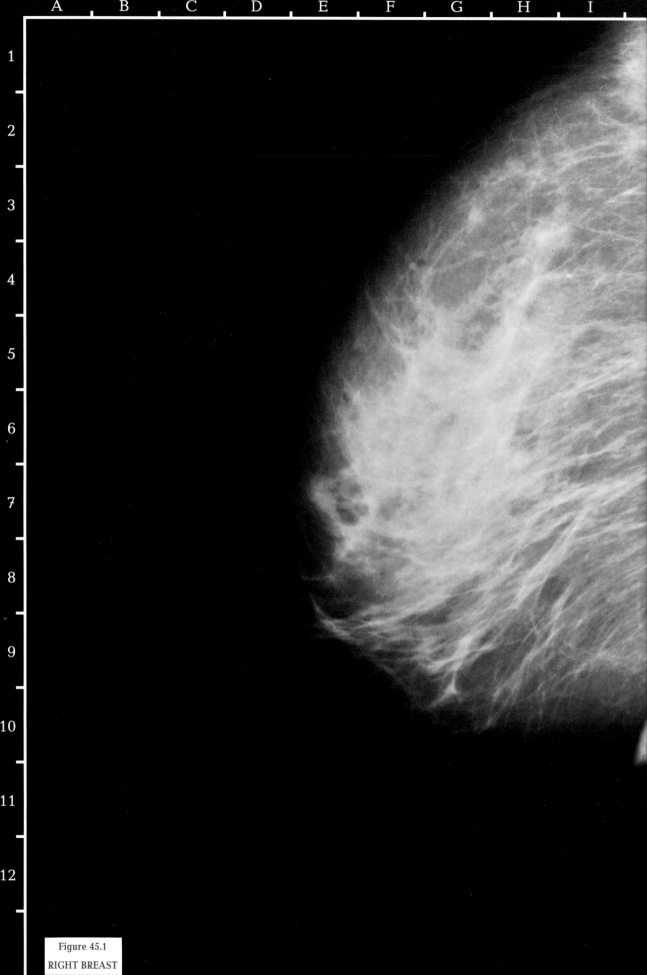

Figure 45.1
RIGHT BREAST

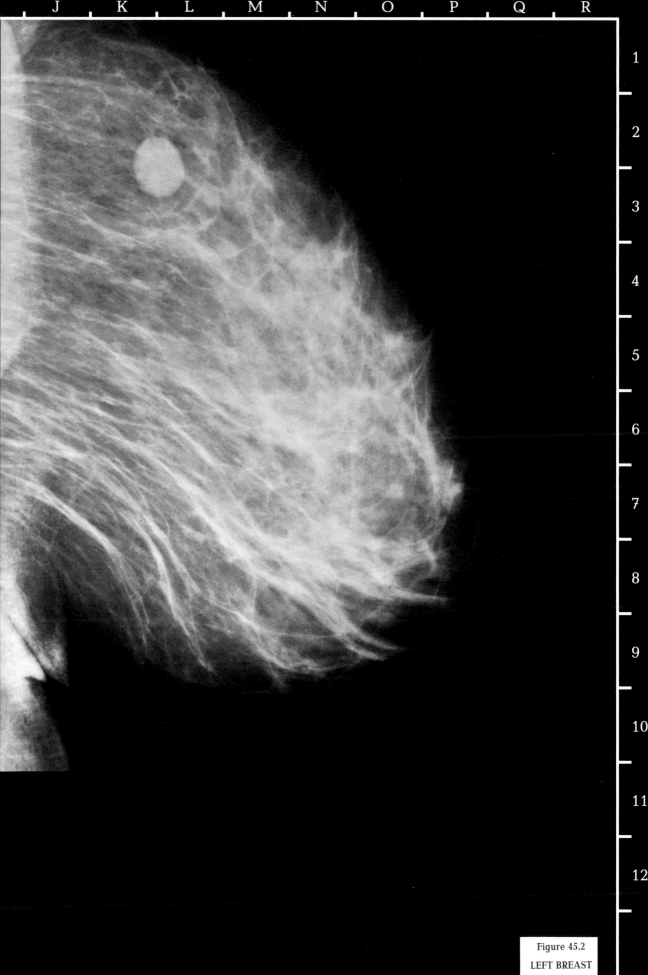

Figure 45.2
LEFT BREAST

Findings

A well-circumscribed 1.5 cm mass (K3) is present in the upper hemisphere of the left breast.

Discussion

In the cephalocaudal mammogram the mass is identified in the left upper–outer quadrant *(Figure 45.3)*. The mediolateral oblique mammograms show enlarged right axillary lymph nodes and a smaller, well-defined mass deep in the upper hemisphere of the right breast as well as the well-defined mass in the left breast *(Figures 45.4 and 45.5)*. The enlarged axillary lymph nodes were soft, movable and slightly tender. Because of their benign mammographic appearance and the presence of axillary adenopathy, the breast masses were felt most likely to represent intramammary lymph nodes.

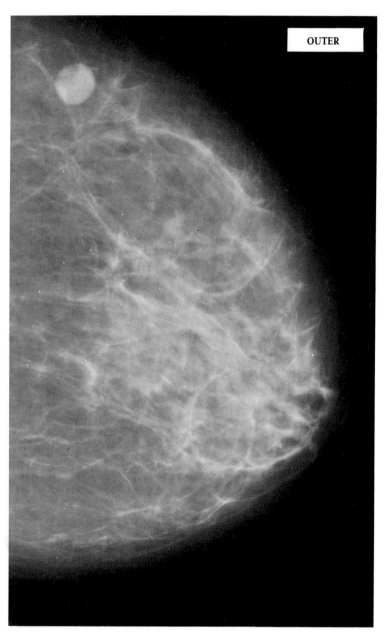

OUTER

Figure 45.3

Cephalocaudal mammogram of left breast shows the well-defined nodule in the outer hemisphere.

Needle-aspiration cytology of the palpable left breast mass revealed atypical reactive lymphoid hyperplasia. A workup resulted in a final diagnosis of lymphoid hyperplasia, secondary to AIDS-related complex.

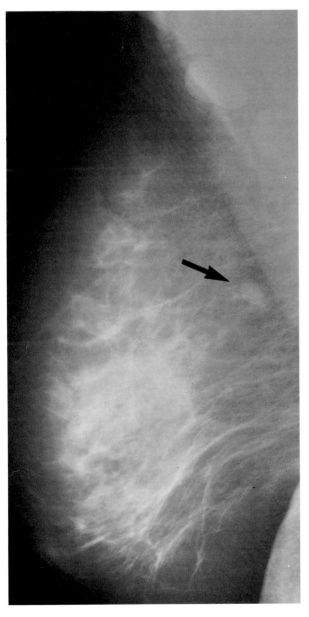

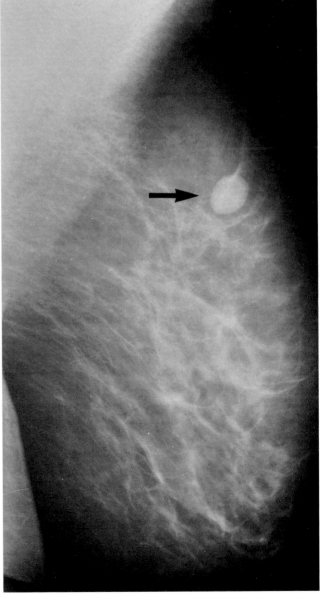

Figure 45.4

Mediolateral oblique view of right breast reveals enlarged axillary lymph nodes and a 1 cm well-circumscribed intramammary nodule (arrow).

Figure 45.5

Mediolateral oblique view of left breast reveals the palpable mass (arrow).

Case 46

This 50-year-old asymptomatic woman was referred for screening mammography.

Films: Right *(Figure 46.1)* and left *(Figure 46.2)* mediolateral oblique mammograms.

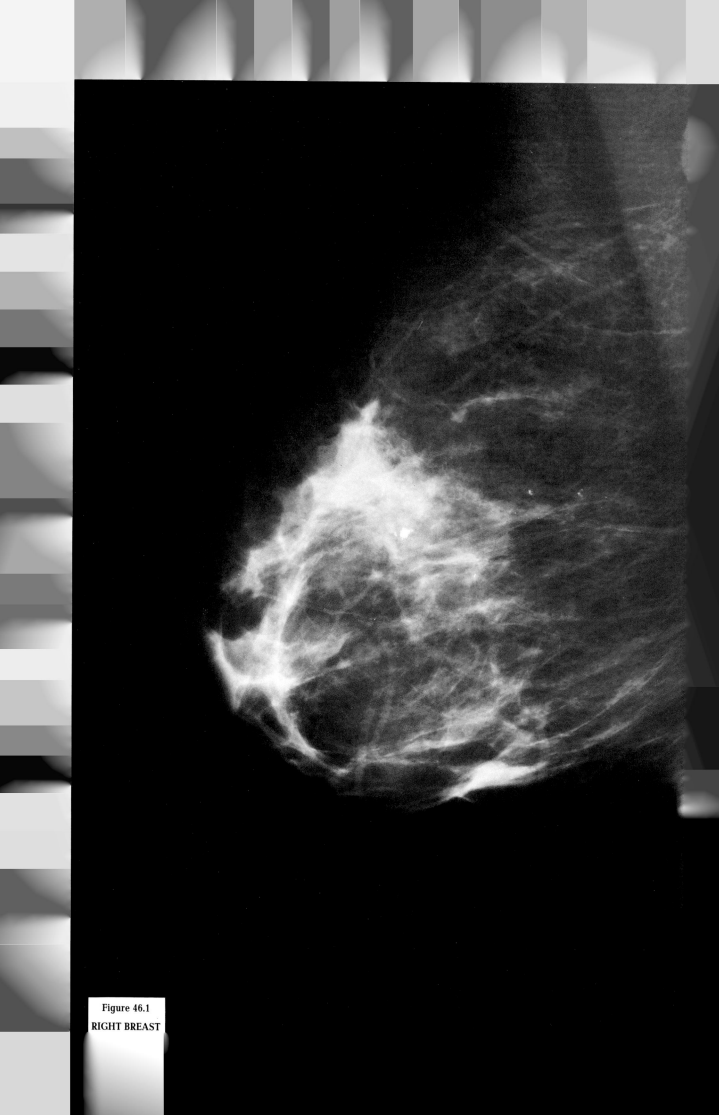

Figure 46.1
RIGHT BREAST

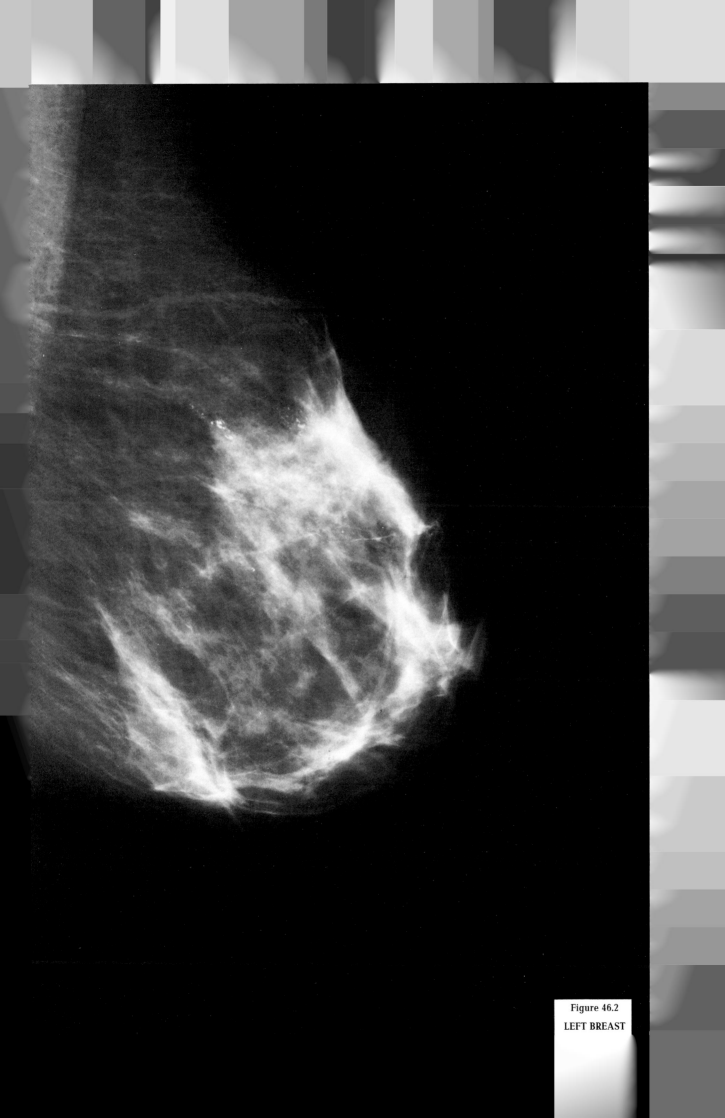

Figure 46.2
LEFT BREAST

Findings

Two clusters with numerous calcifications are present in the left breast (L5, M5), and one cluster with numerous calcifications is present on the right (H6).

Discussion

The calcifications in the three clusters are numerous, varying in size and shape, and some have configurations that suggest a location within the ducts *(Figures 46.3 and 46.4)*. Thus, multifocal carcinoma has to be considered a diagnostic possibility. In order to minimize surgical biopsy deformities, each of the three clusters was localized with a needle-hookwire system prior to biopsy *(Figures 46.5 and 46.6)*. Biopsy revealed that all three clusters represented fibrocystic changes, including fibrosis, apocrine metaplasia and microcysts.

This case represents a false-positive mammogram that led to unnecessary biopsies. Clustered

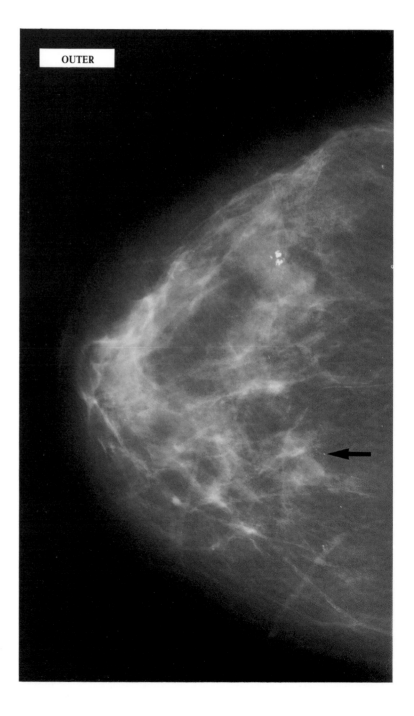

Figure 46.3

Cephalocaudal mammogram of the right breast. The clustered calcifications (arrow) are barely visible.

benign calcifications are the most common cause for a false-positive mammogram. There has been considerable debate over what should be considered the most appropriate true-positive rate for screening.[21] True-positive biopsy rates as low as 10 percent (1 cancer detected for every 10 biopsies) and as high as 40 percent have been advocated, with more early cancers detected in the more aggressive setting where more biopsies are done.[56] To help radiologists determine whether their biopsy rate is acceptable in the setting of their own practices and in comparison to others, they are encouraged to keep track of the results of the biopsies resulting from their screening mammograms.[99] In our practice only 1 in 3–5 biopsies performed by our surgeons for palpable breast masses is positive for malignancy, and these palpable cancers have a less favorable prognosis than the earlier nonpalpable lesions detected by mammography.

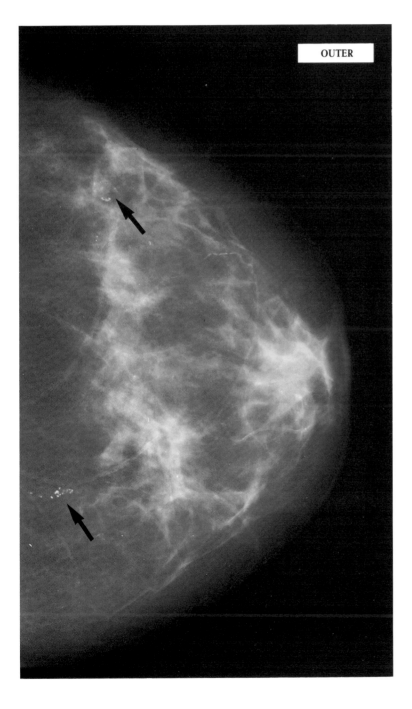

Figure 46.4

Cephalocaudal mammogram of the left breast. The two clusters (arrows) are widely separated.

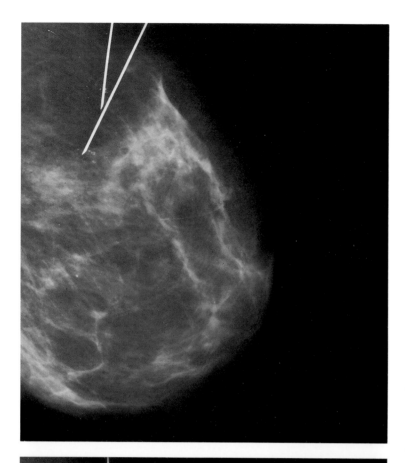

Figure 46.5

Lateral mammogram at the time of prebiopsy needle localization. Two needles have been placed, one at each of the clusters.

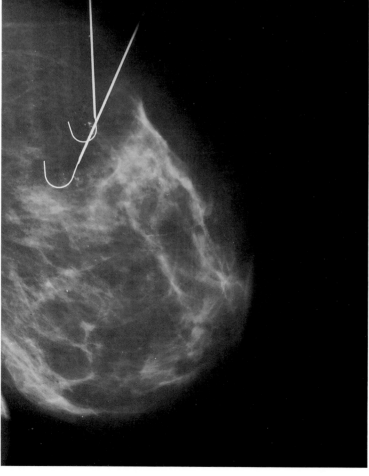

Figure 46.6

J-wires have been afterloaded through the needles. The hook anchors the needle in place when the patient is transported to surgery.

Case 47

This 37-year-old woman was referred for an abnormality found on screening mammography.

Films: Right *(Figure 47.1)* and left *(Figure 47.2)* mediolateral oblique mammograms.

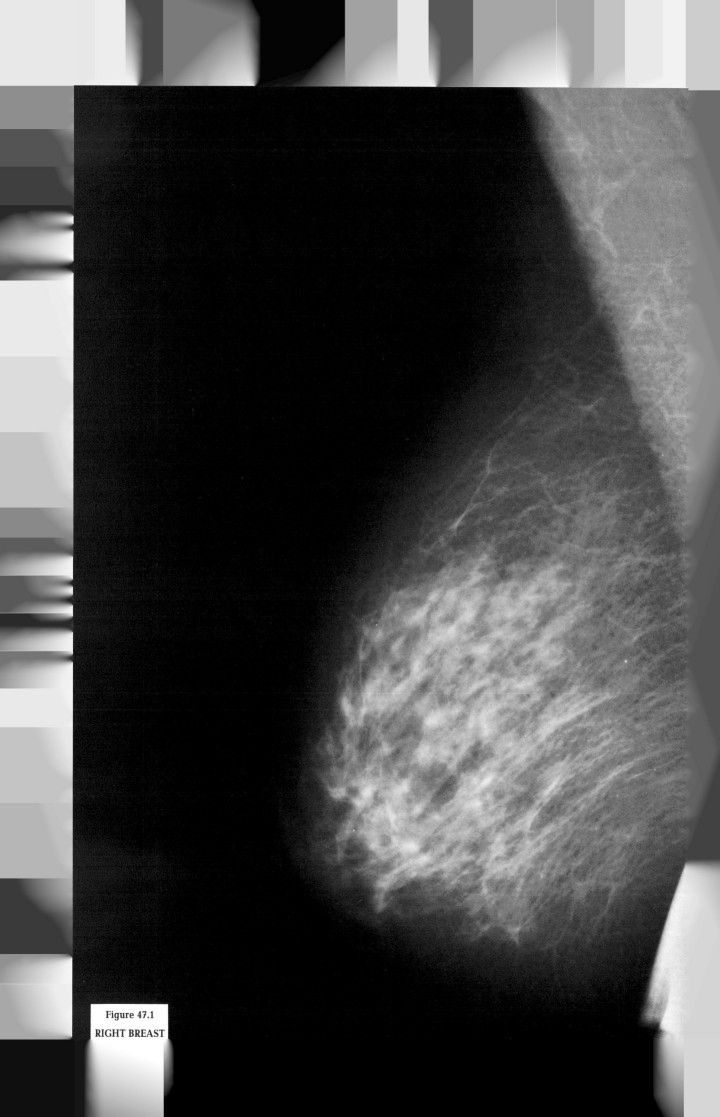

Figure 47.1
RIGHT BREAST

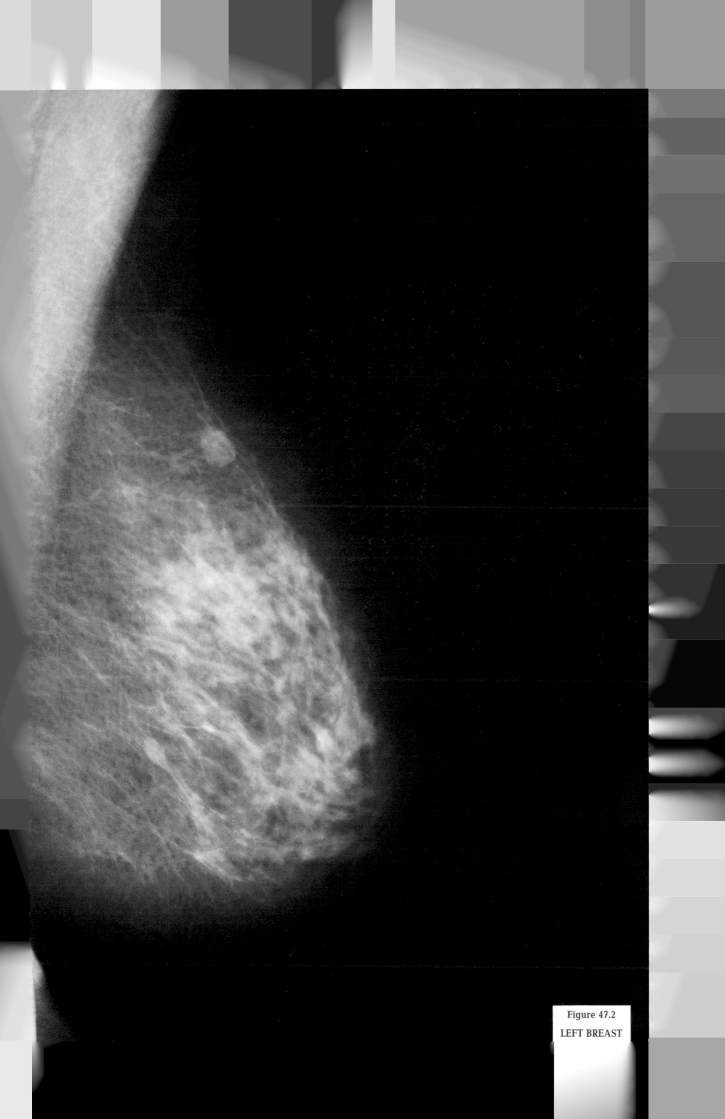

Figure 47.2
LEFT BREAST

Findings

There is a prominent ductal pattern in both breasts. A 1 cm well-defined oval nodule is present in the upper hemisphere of the left breast (L5).

Discussion

The nodule has a sharp margin and central radiolucency. In the cephalocaudal view, it is located in the outer hemisphere *(Figure 47.3)*. The well-defined margin is confirmed in a spot-

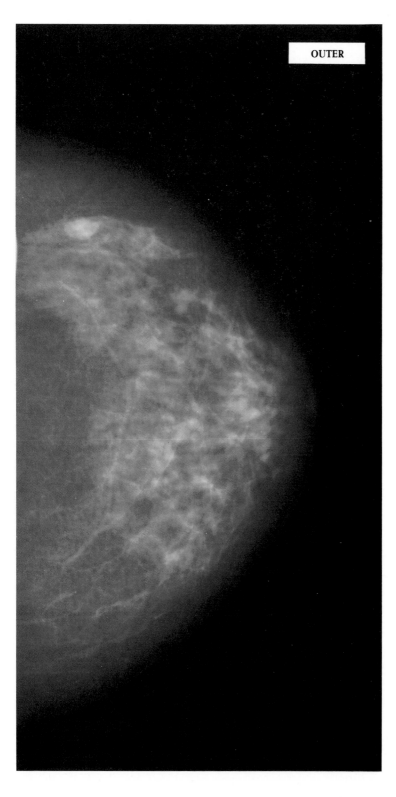

OUTER

Figure 47.3

Cephalocaudal mammogram shows the nodule in the outer hemisphere.

compression view *(Figure 47.4)*. The nodule's location in the upper–outer quadrant, its well-defined margins and its central lucency are characteristic of an intramammary lymph node.[38] Although biopsy was not recommended, the patient insisted on having the nodule removed because she had been told that it was suspicious for malignancy at the time of the original mammograms.

Biopsy showed a lymph node containing benign reactive hyperplasia *(Figure 47.5 and Figure 47.6)*. Regional or systemic immune responses may cause lymph nodes to enlarge.

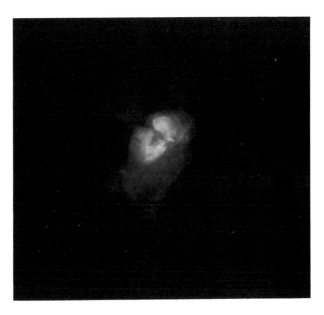

Figure 47.5

Specimen radiography verifies that the lesion has been excised and shows its radiolucent center.

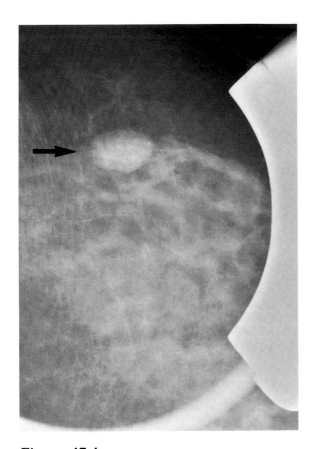

Figure 47.4

Spot-compression view shows a well-defined margin throughout the boundary of the lesion (arrow).

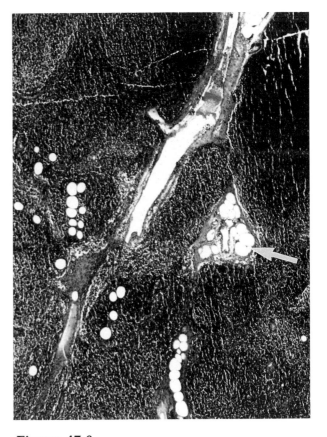

Figure 47.6

Low-power histologic section. Reactive hyperplasia of lymph node. The fat (arrow) in the center is responsible for the central radiolucency seen in the mammogram.

Case 48

This 70-year-old woman was referred for a lump in her left breast. She had had generalized non-Hodgkin's lymphoma for 3 years.

Films: Right *(Figure 48.1)* and left *(Figure 48.2)* mediolateral mammograms.

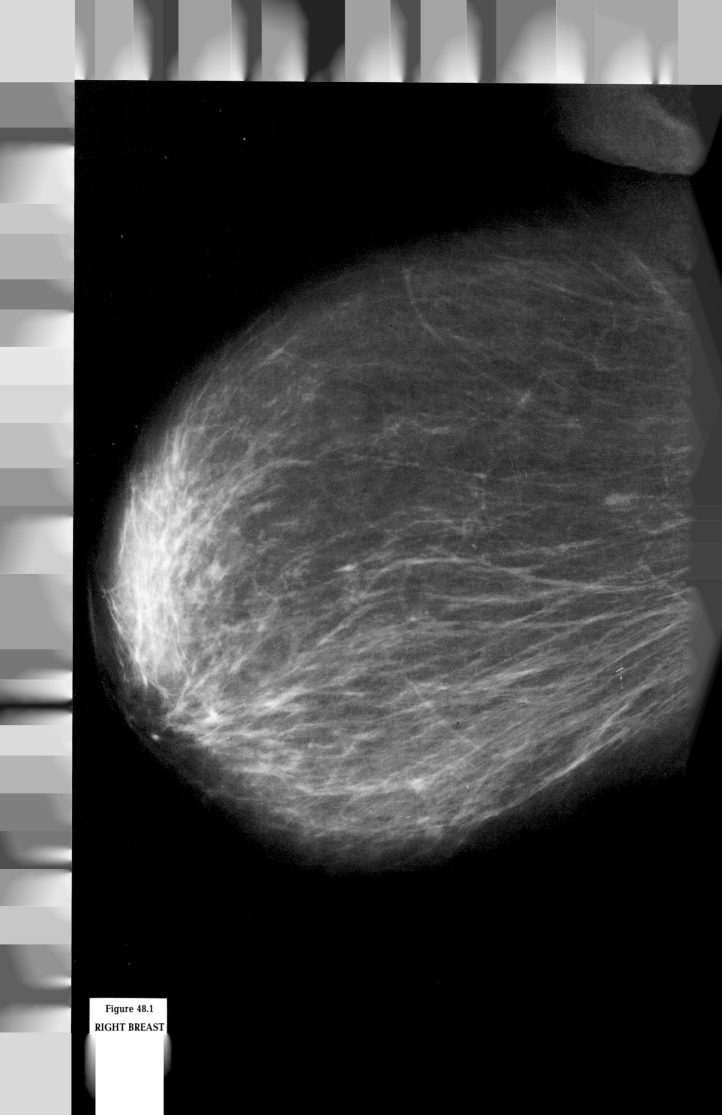

Figure 48.1
RIGHT BREAST

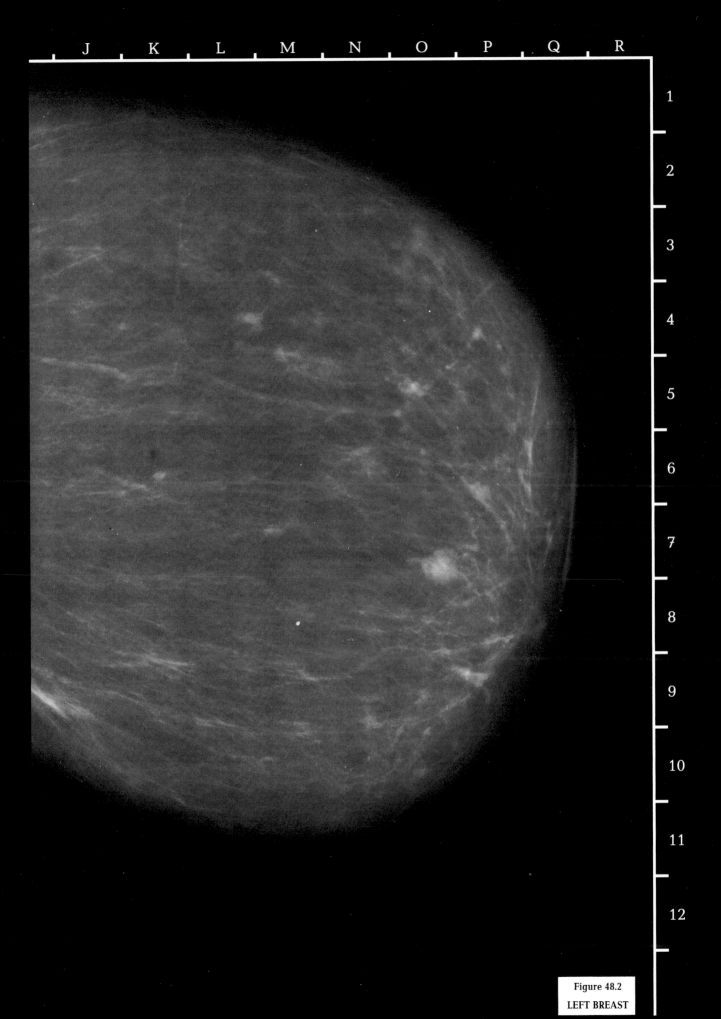

Figure 48.2
LEFT BREAST

Findings

The breasts are large and fatty and contain bilateral nodules. One of the nodules in the left breast is larger than the others (P8), and matches the site of the palpable abnormality.

Discussion

The margins of the oval density are indistinct *(Figure 48.3)*. A biopsy was recommended to rule out malignancy. The biopsy revealed a focus of non-Hodgkin's lymphoma *(Figure 48.4)*.

Metastases to the breast may arise from any extramammary primary tumor. The reported autopsy incidence of metastasis to the breast from malignant neoplasms other than breast carcinoma varies from 1.7 to 6.6 percent.[1,55,122] Due to its late presentation in the course of malignant disease, a metastatic breast nodule is rarely the initial sign of malignancy. Metastatic nodules may be multiple or solitary, but most often are solitary when first detected.[20] They are most frequently found in the upper–outer quadrant. Characteristically, the margin is either relatively well defined or only moderately infiltrative. The most common metastases are from malignant melanoma, but a wide variety of other tumors may secondarily involve the breast.[147]

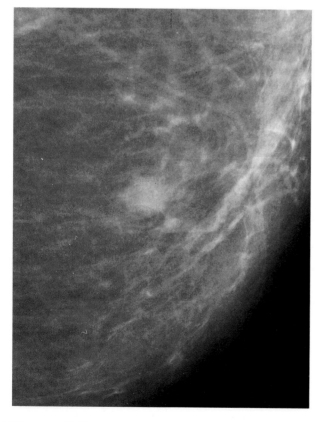

Figure 48.3

Close-up of lesion shows relatively poorly defined margins.

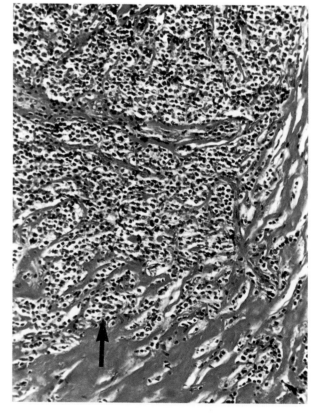

Figure 48.4

Low-power histologic section. The mass consists of atypical lymphocytes (arrow) infiltrating the surrounding breast tissue. **Diagnosis**: Lymphoma.

Case 49

This 77-year-old woman had a left mastectomy for invasive lobular carcinoma 14 years ago. Ten years ago she had a biopsy of the upper–outer quadrant of the right breast which disclosed benign intraductal papillomatosis. She was referred for routine follow-up mammograms.

Films: Right mediolateral oblique *(Figure 49.1)* and cephalocaudal *(Figure 49.2)* mammograms.

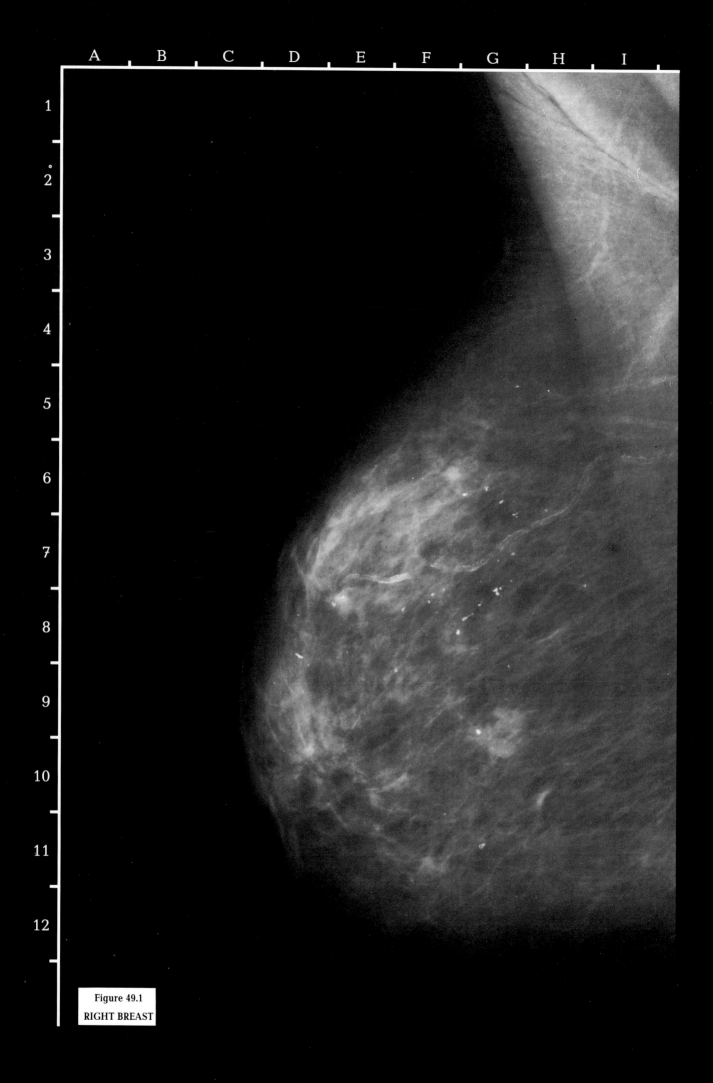

Figure 49.1
RIGHT BREAST

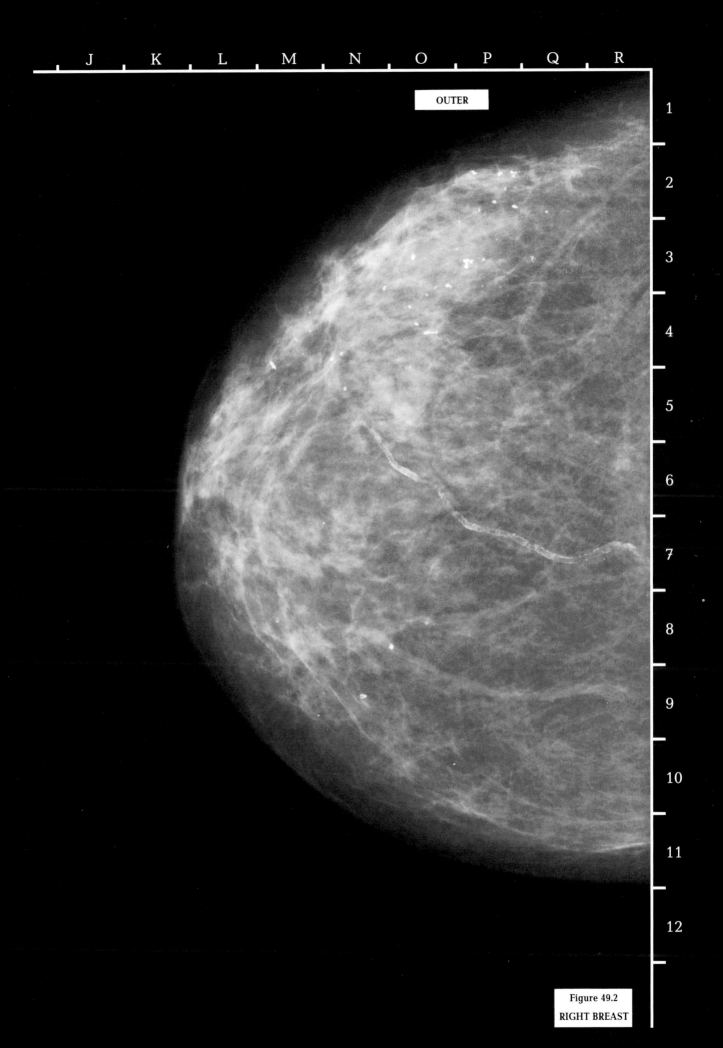

J K L M N O P Q R

OUTER

1
2
3
4
5
6
7
8
9
10
11
12

Figure 49.2
RIGHT BREAST

Findings

In the oblique view, there is an indentation of the skin (D7). Calcifications are present in the upper–outer quadrant. In addition, the oblique view shows a vague density (G9) posterior to the nipple, which is not identified in the cephalocaudal view.

Discussion

The skin indentation noted on the oblique view matches the site of previous surgery. The calcifica-

tions are coarse, and some show lucent centers, findings typical of benign secretory calcifications. The calcifications were present in previous mammograms and had not changed.

The density observed in the oblique view, but not the cephalocaudal, was thought to represent a superimposition of normal tissues. Physical examination failed to reveal any palpable abnormality at this site. However, because of the patient's history of previous carcinoma, a 6-month follow-up examination was recommended.

The follow-up oblique view (Figure 49.3) shows an increase in the size and density of the lesion

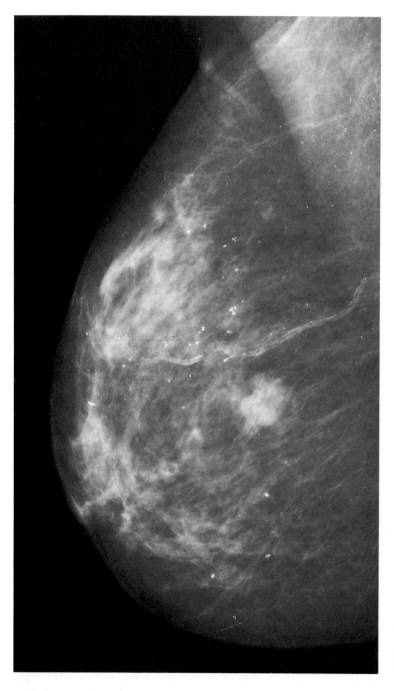

Figure 49.3

Six-month follow-up mediolateral oblique view. The lesion is larger and denser.

which is now also discernible in the cephalocaudal view *(Figure 49.4)*. A lateral mammogram localized the lesion to the lower hemisphere *(Figure 49.5)*. A biopsy revealed infiltrating lobular carcinoma.

Patients with a history of breast carcinoma have a higher risk for development of a second breast carcinoma than women in the general population. The risk for development of a contralateral carcinoma after mastectomy has been reported to be 1 percent per year after mastectomy.[118] This risk of subsequent carcinoma in the contralateral breast varies with age at time of diagnosis, with women less than 40 years of age having a 3-times greater risk of bilaterality than older women.[24] Lobular carcinoma has an even higher incidence of bilaterality than ductal carcinoma.[35]

This case illustrates the value of a follow-up examination for equivocal findings when a biopsy is not performed. Usually such a follow-up is performed at 4–6 months, and if there is no change the patient is followed annually for at least 2 more years.[64]

When one localizes a nonpalpable lesion detected on a two-view oblique-cephalocaudal examination, it is important to perform a true

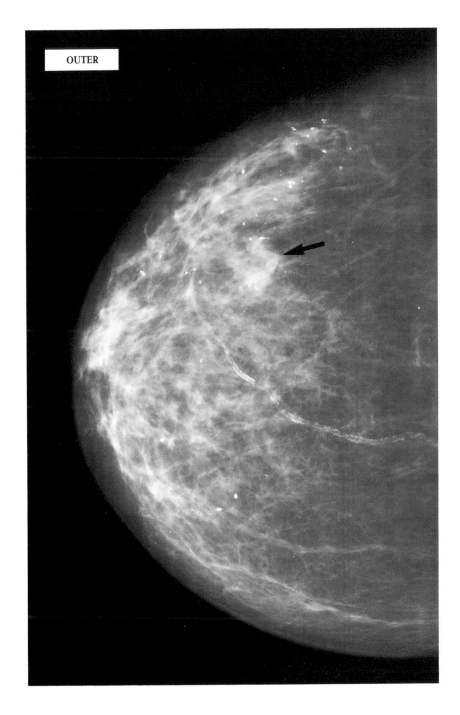

OUTER

Figure 49.4

Cephalocaudal view. The lesion (arrow) is present in the outer hemisphere.

lateral view prior to needle placement, since determination of the exact location requires two views at right angles. In this case, the lateral view identified the true location of the lesion—in the lower hemisphere *(Figure 49.5)*—whereas it appeared to be in the upper hemisphere in the oblique projection *(Figure 49.3)*.

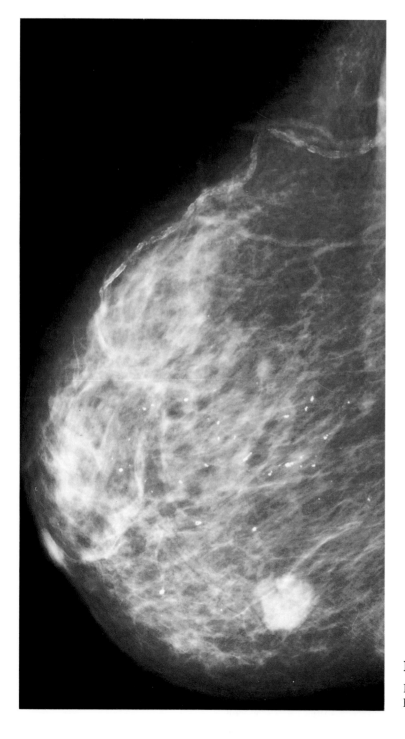

Figure 49.5

Lateral view. The lesion is in the lower hemisphere.

Case 50

This 54-year-old woman was referred for screening mammography.

Films: Right *(Figure 50.1)* and left *(Figure 50.2)* mediolateral oblique mammograms.

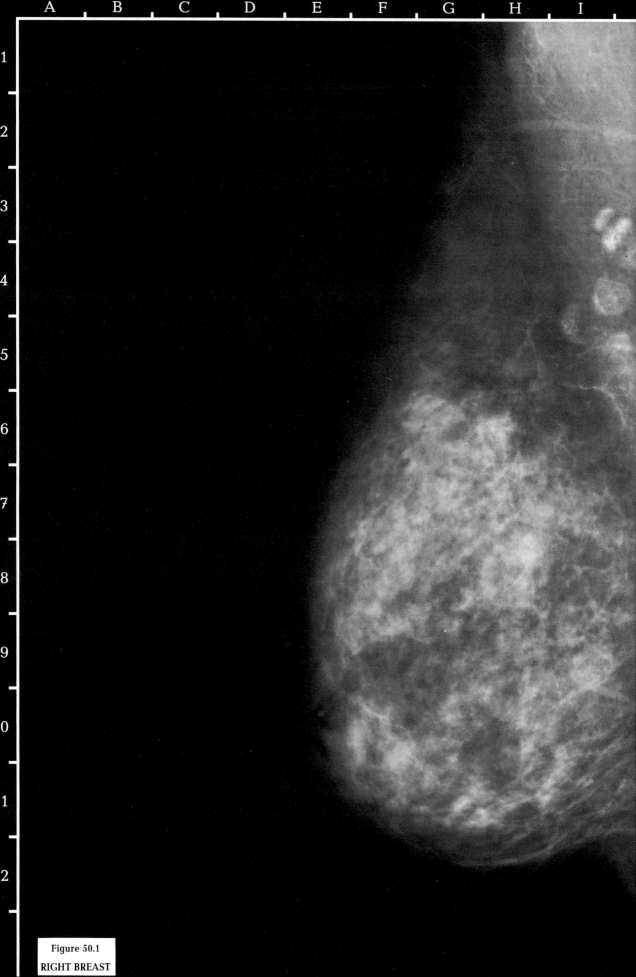

Figure 50.1
RIGHT BREAST

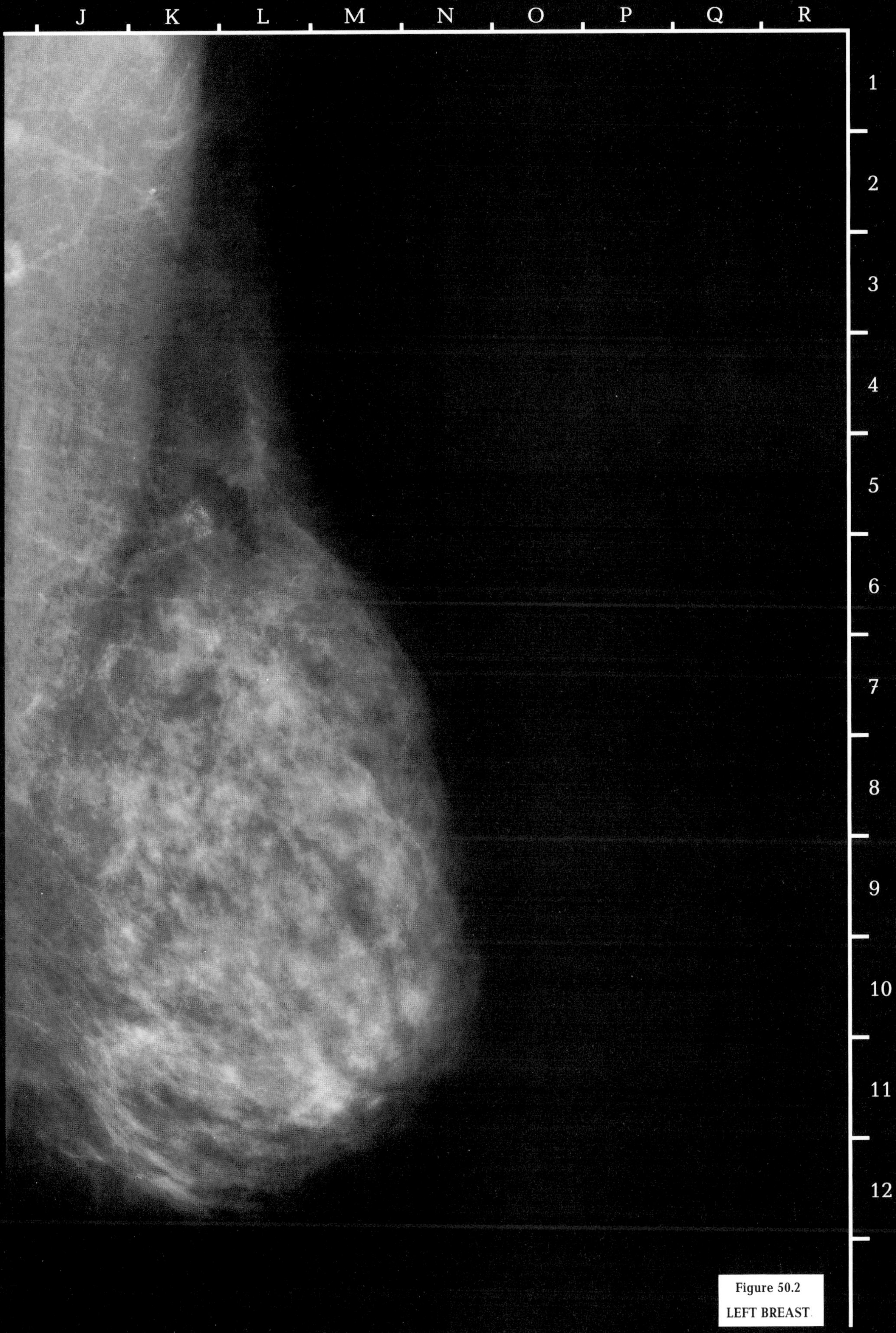

J K L M N O P Q R

1
2
3
4
5
6
7
8
9
10
11
12

Figure 50.2
LEFT BREAST

Findings

The breasts are dense. There are punctate calcifications in the axillary lymph nodes on the right. In the left breast a cluster of calcifications (K5) is present at the base of the axillary tail.

Discussion

Exaggerated lateral positioning for the left cephalocaudal mammogram reveals punctate calcifications in the outer part of the breast *(Figures 50.3, 50.4 and 50.5).* In this case, the clue to the diagnosis resides in the patient's history: she had a long history of gold therapy for rheumatoid arthritis. The apparent 'calcifications' are in axillary and intramammary lymph nodes, and actually represent deposits of gold.[9,22] The patient has been followed for 6 years without change in the mammograms. It is rare for mammograms to depict calcifications in nodal metastases.

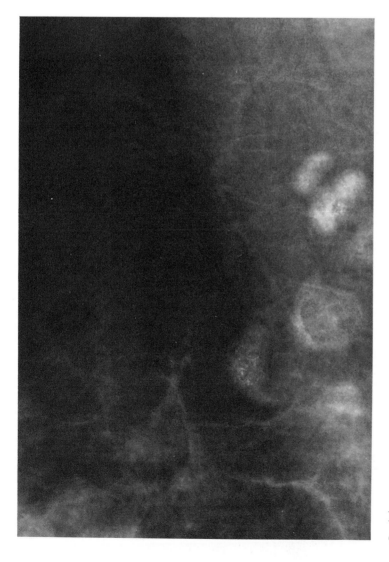

Figure 50.3

Close-up of right axillary lymph nodes.

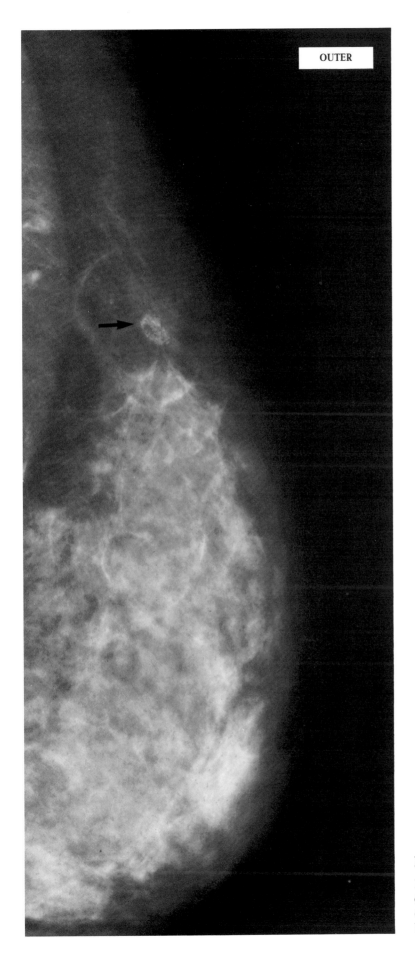

Figure 50.4

Left cephalocaudal mammogram, exaggerated outer positioning. The calcific deposits (arrow) are in the outer breast, at the base of the axillary tail.

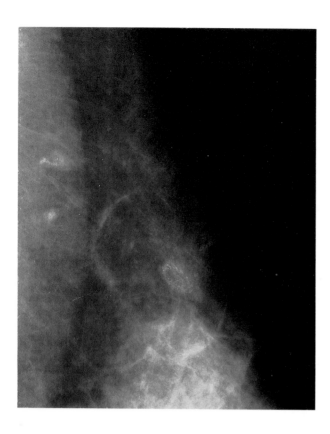

Figure 50.5

Close-up of left intramammary lymph node.

Case 51

This 28-year-old woman had a 3-month history of increasing tenderness in her left breast.

Films: Right *(Figure 51.1)* and left *(Figure 51.2)* mediolateral oblique mammograms.

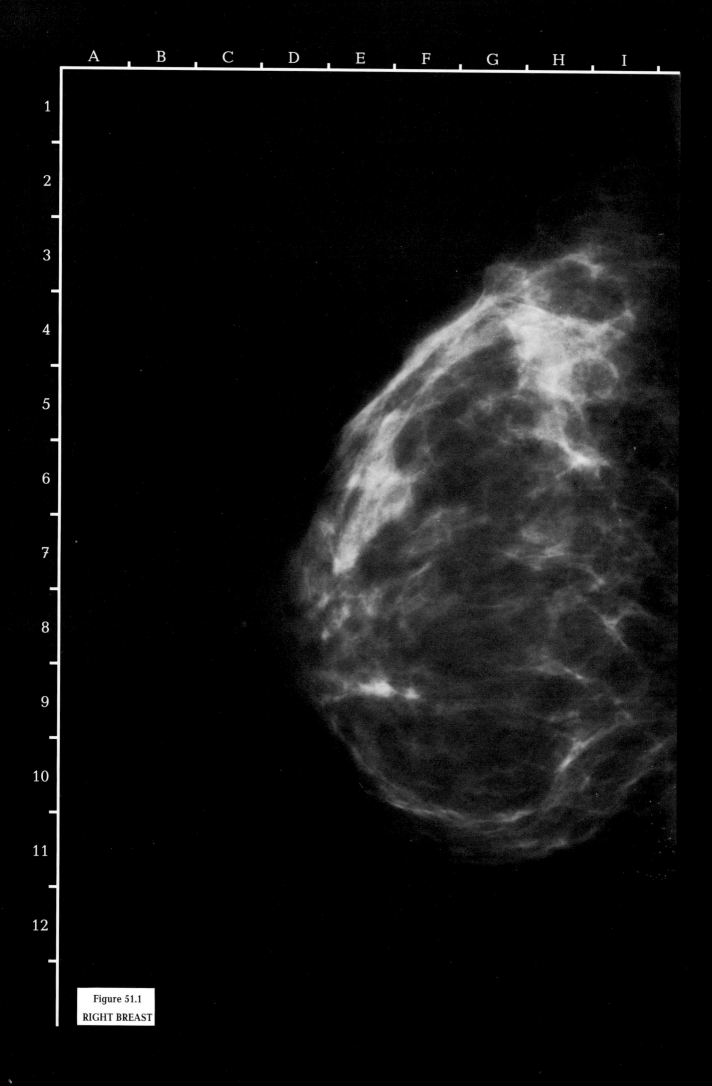

Figure 51.1
RIGHT BREAST

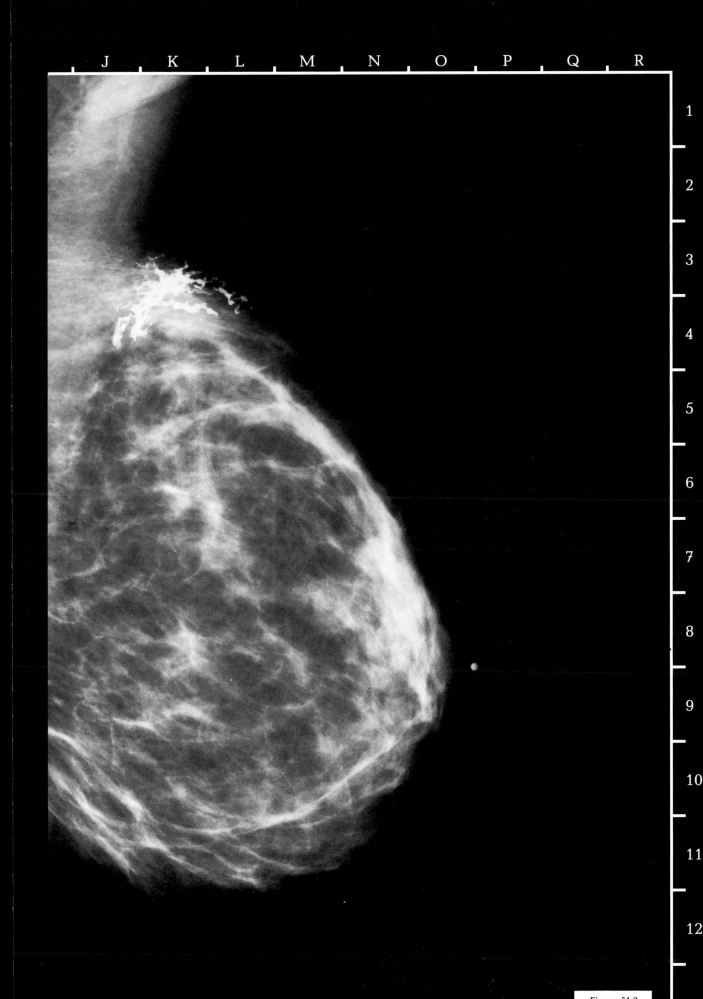

Figure 51.2
LEFT BREAST

Findings

Metal markers (beebees) identify the nipples. Tortuous tubular calcifications (K4) are present in the upper–outer quadrant of the left breast.

Discussion

The calcified tubular structures are too large to be ducts this far from the nipple. Some of the calcified structures are immediately below the skin *(Figure 51.3)*. They do not have the parallel railroad-track appearance of arterial calcifications. The calcifications fill the lumens of structures with an appearance most consistent with dilated, tortuous veins. The clinical history and radiographic findings are consistent with calcified venous thrombi resulting from Mondor's disease, or superficial thrombophlebitis of the thoracoepigastric veins overlying the breast.[53,62,143] This benign condition may be clinically evident when it involves veins in the subcutaneous tissue of the breast. The earliest symptoms are tenderness, pain and redness in the region of the involved vein. Typically, the condition progresses to swelling, a sense of tightness and the development of a cord-like lesion of varying length. If the inflammatory reaction provokes retraction of the overlying skin, it may be confused clinically with carcinoma. The condition is self-limited and the symptoms resolve without treatment, generally in a few weeks. Radiographically, the thrombosed veins are usually characterized by thickened subcutaneous cords in one projection. Calcification of the involved veins is unusual.

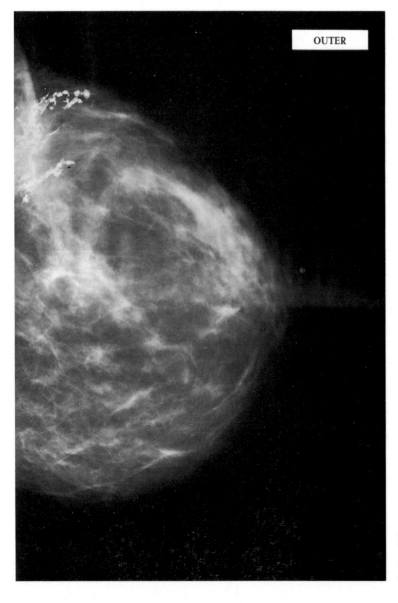

OUTER

Figure 51.3

Cephalocaudal projection. The coarse calcifications are tortuous and branching.

Case 52

This 60-year-old woman was referred because of an abnormal screening mammogram.

Films: Right *(Figure 52.1)* and left *(Figure 52.2)* mediolateral oblique mammograms.

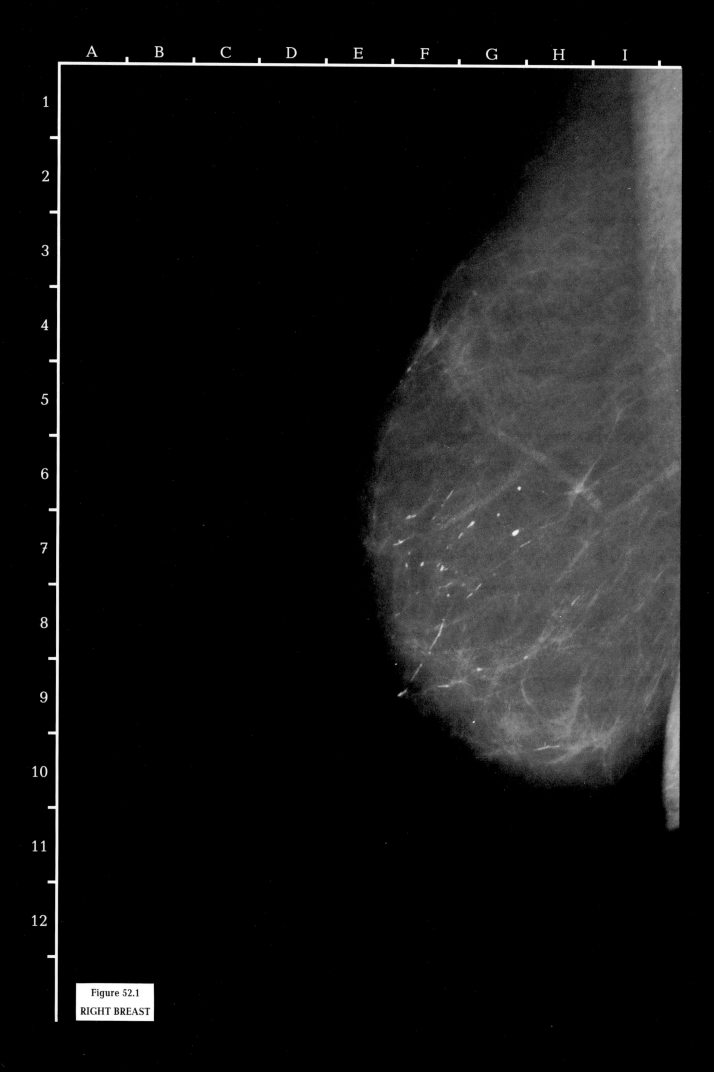

Figure 52.1
RIGHT BREAST

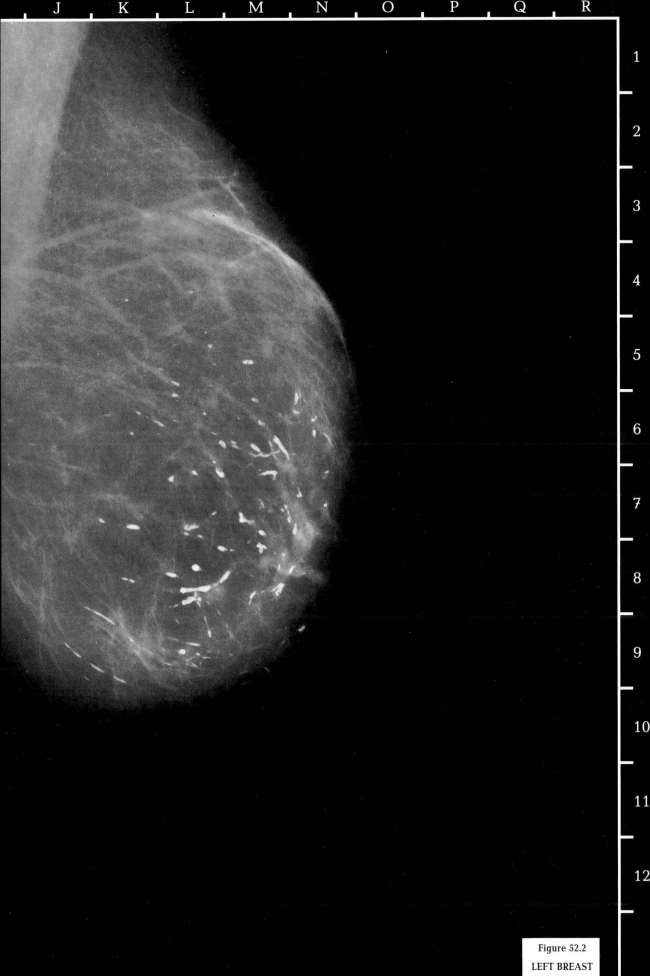

Figure 52.2
LEFT BREAST

Findings

There are bilateral coarse linear calcifications. In the left subareolar area are several prominent ducts and a 6 mm nodular density (N8).

Discussion

The calcifications are typical for secretory disease, or mammary duct ectasia. In this condition, the ducts contain coarse, solid linear and ring-like calcifications of inspissated intraluminal contents, and may be surrounded by periductal fibrosis. A biopsy was recommended for the nodular density, which was felt to be particularly suspicious because of the associated ductal thickening. The biopsy revealed only mammary duct ectasia (Figure 52.3).

Mammary duct ectasia is characterized by inspissated secretions, dilated ducts, and a chronic interstitial inflammatory reaction. It occurs most often in peri- or postmenopausal women.[54] Its etiology is not certain, but may be related to the accumulation of thickened secretions within the ducts that leads to dilatation and rupture of the duct wall. Leakage of the secretions into the surrounding tissue results in a chronic inflammatory response often containing many plasma cells. 'Obliterative mastitis', 'plasma cell mastitis' and 'subareolar fibrosis' are terms applied to the late stages of this disease. Patients may present with a focal or ill-defined area of pain, tenderness, induration and ropiness in the peri- or subareolar region. Fixation to the skin, with retraction of the skin or nipple, or the presence of nipple discharge may cause the lesion to be mistaken for neoplasm.

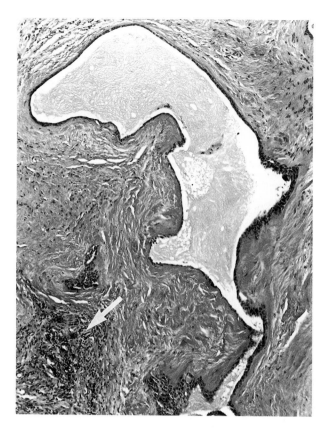

Figure 52.3

A dilated duct is seen filled with inspissated secretions, and surrounded by periductal inflammation (arrow) and fibrosis. **Diagnosis**: Mammary duct ectasia.

The majority of women are asymptomatic, with the mammographic calcifications the only manifestation of the disease. There is no predisposition to breast cancer.[33]

Case 53

This 60-year-old woman was referred because of an abnormality in the upper–outer quadrant of the left breast found on a routine screening mammogram.

Films: Left mediolateral *(Figure 53.1)* and exaggerated outer cephalocaudal views *(Figure 53.2)*.

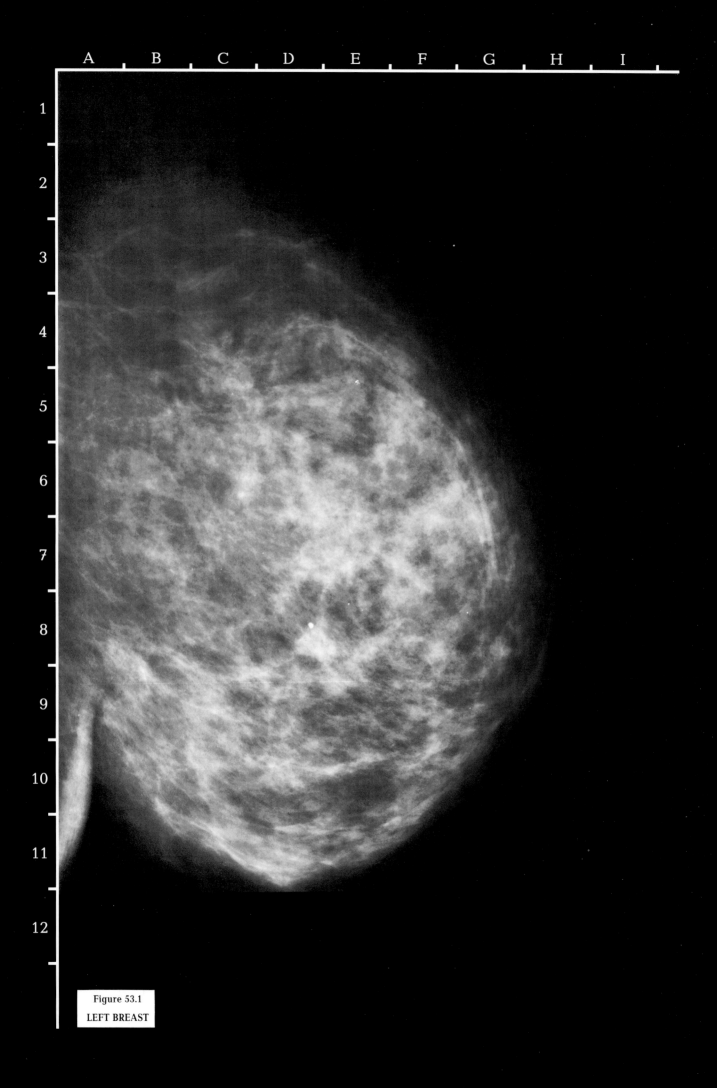

Figure 53.1
LEFT BREAST

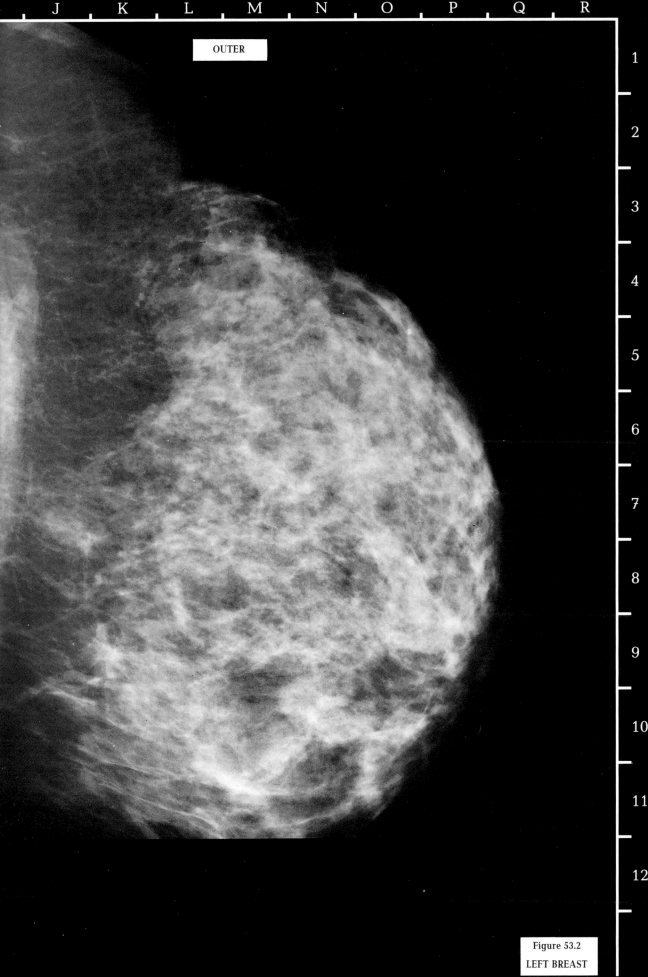

OUTER

J K L M N O P Q R

1
2
3
4
5
6
7
8
9
10
11
12

Figure 53.2
LEFT BREAST

Findings

A cluster of calcifications is barely visible in the upper–outer quadrant of the left breast (C5), (M4), in association with mild-to-moderate architectural distortion of the surrounding tissue. On the lateral view is a solitary calcification and a 1 cm density inferior to it (E8).

Discussion

Spot-magnification views of the 1 cm density seen in the lateral view failed to confirm the presence of a mass *(Figure 53.3)*. Therefore, a biopsy was recommended only for the cluster of calcifications in the upper–outer quadrant. In the radiograph of the excised specimen, the calcifications and the architectural distortion are more obvious than in the original mammogram *(Figure 53.4)*. Histologic examination revealed tubular carcinoma *(Figure 53.5)*.

The average age of women with tubular carcinoma is 53 years.[54] It is one of the well-differentiated, least-frequent types of carcinoma of the breast.[43] A pure tubular carcinoma rarely metastasizes. However, when it coexists with another type of carcinoma, the extent of the latter determines the overall prognosis.[109]

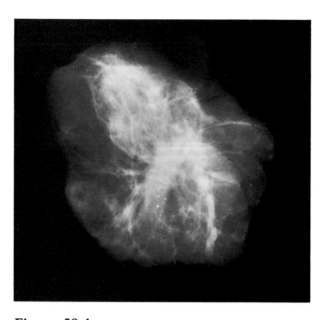

Figure 53.4

Specimen radiograph.

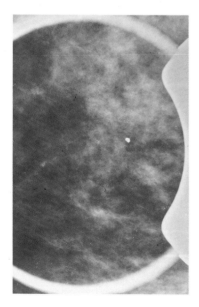

Figure 53.3

Spot-magnification view. The solitary calcification is seen, but no mass.

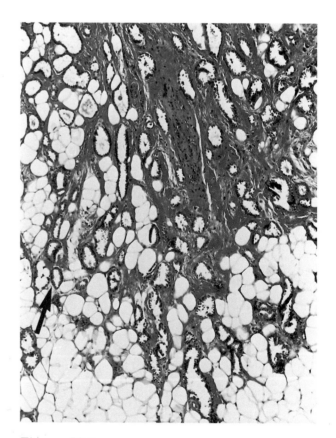

Figure 53.5

Low-power histologic section. The tumor consists of tubules (arrow) within a fibrous stroma, invading surrounding mammary fat. **Diagnosis**: Tubular carcinoma.

Case 54

This 65-year-old woman was referred for screening mammography.

Films: Right *(Figure 54.1)* and left *(Figure 54.2)* mediolateral oblique mammograms.

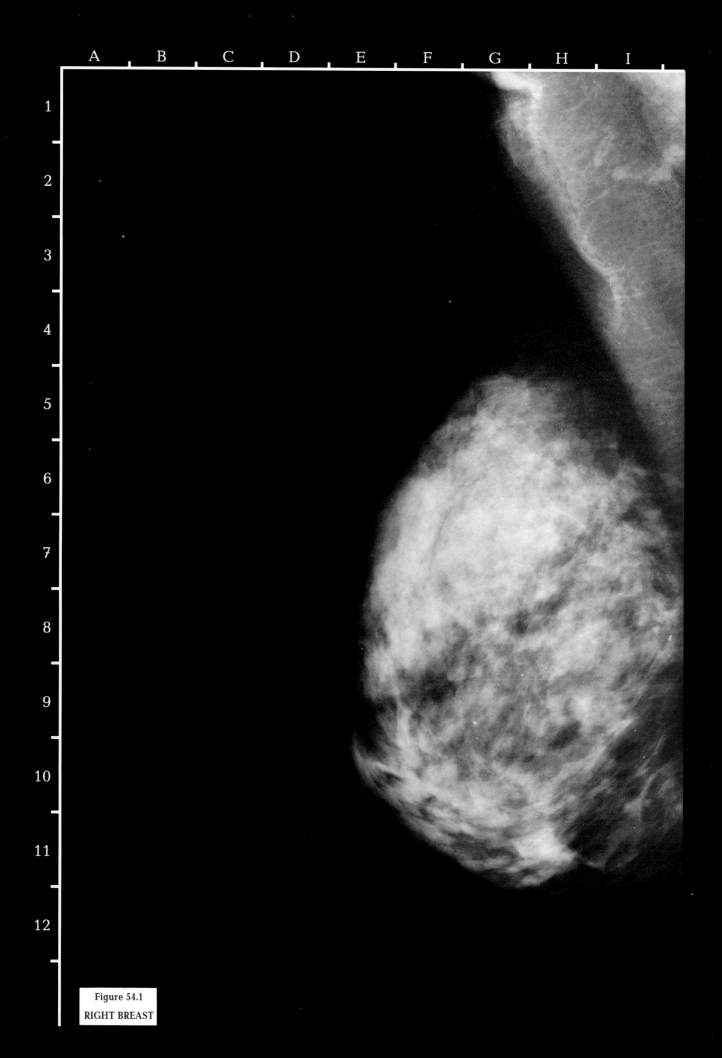

Figure 54.1
RIGHT BREAST

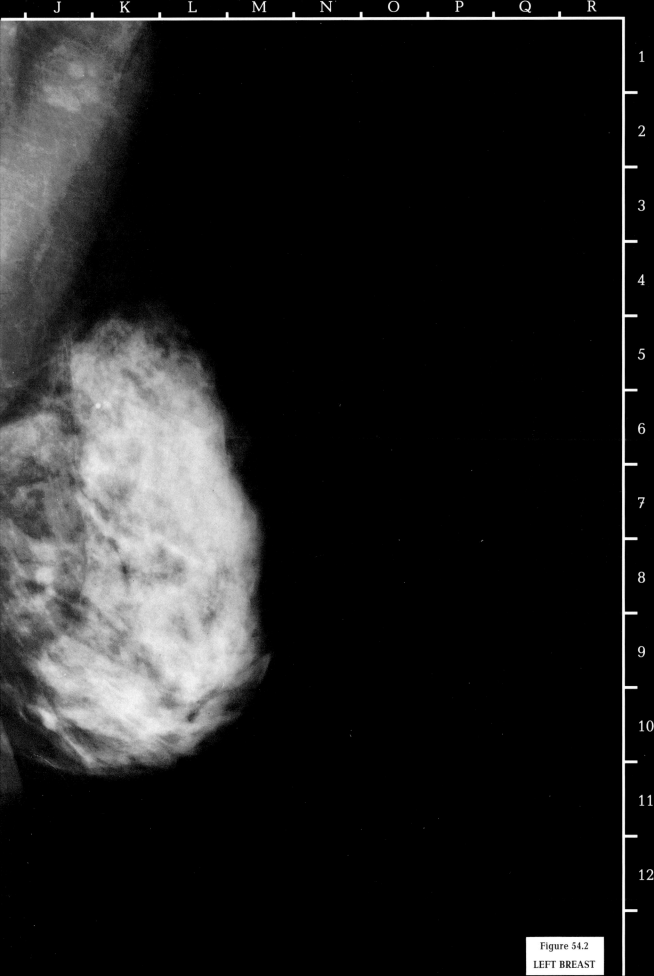

Figure 54.2
LEFT BREAST

Findings

There are several benign solitary calcifications. A barely visible cluster of 5 calcifications is present in the upper hemisphere of the right breast (G5). Benign-appearing lymph nodes are present in both axillae.

Discussion

The breasts are unusually dense for a 65-year-old woman. The small cluster of calcifications in the upper hemisphere of the right breast *(Figure 54.3)* was not seen on the routine cephalocaudal projection *(Figure 54.4)*. Therefore, exaggerated cephalocaudal views were performed, and they

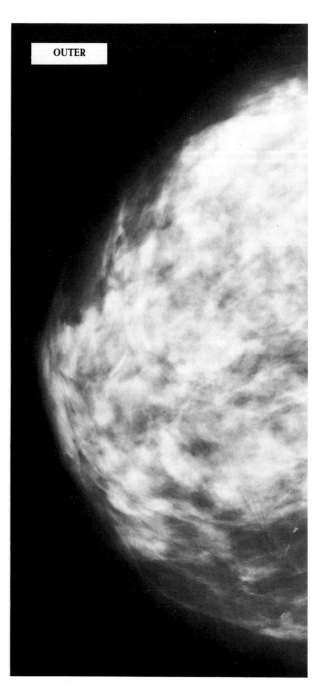

Figure 54.4

Routine cephalocaudal projection does not show the calcifications.

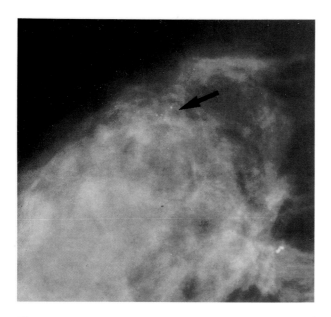

Figure 54.3

Close-up of calcifications (arrow).

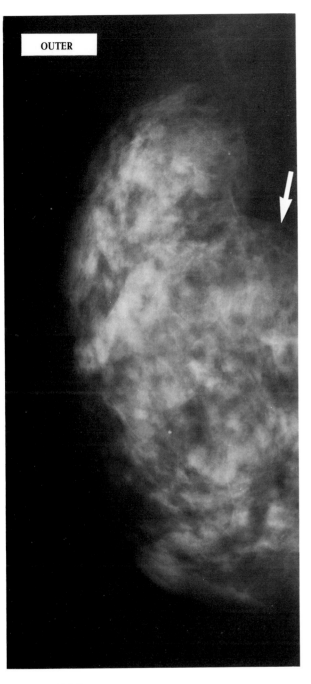

depicted the calcifications deep in the outer hemisphere *(Figure 54.5)*. The calcifications were not visible in mammograms performed 1 year earlier. A biopsy was recommended. Under mammographic guidance, a hookwire was placed so that its tip was at the calcifications. The surgeon found a small mass near the tip of the hookwire *(Figure 54.6)*. Histological sections revealed both lobular carcinoma in situ *(Figure 54.7)* and invasive lobular carcinoma *(Figure 54.8)*.

This case illustrates the difficulty of identification of a small mass within a dense breast. The biopsy was performed only because of the presence of the calcifications. The patient must be followed closely because lobular carcinoma has a high incidence of multicentricity and bilaterality.[35]

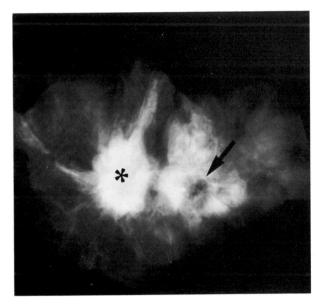

Figure 54.5

Exaggerated outer cephalocaudal view. The calcifications (arrow) are located deep in the outer breast.

Figure 54.6

Specimen radiograph. A dense spiculated mass (asterisk) lies adjacent to the calcifications (arrow).

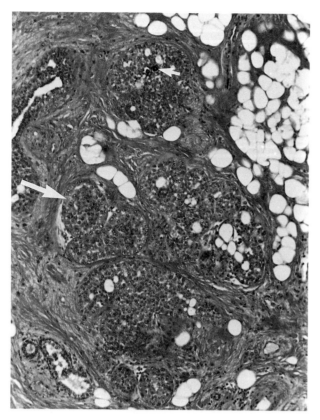

Figure 54.7

Low-power histologic section. The lobules (large arrow) and ductules are filled with malignant cells. Calcifications (small arrow) are seen within some of the lobules. **Diagnosis**: Lobular carcinoma in situ.

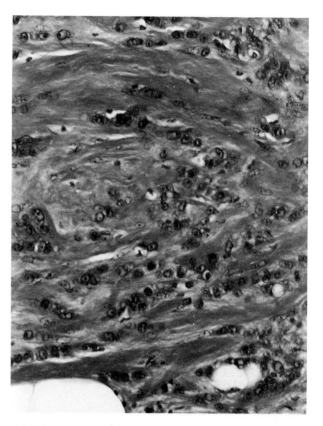

Figure 54.8

Low-power histologic section. Infiltrating lobular carcinoma characterized by small nests and single files of cells ('indian files') embedded within a dense fibrous stroma. **Diagnosis**: Invasive lobular carcinoma.

References

1 Abrams HL, Spiro R, Goldstein N, Metastases in carcinoma: an analysis of 1000 autopsied cases, *Cancer* (1950) **3**:74–85.

2 Adair FE, Munzer JT, Fat necrosis of the female breast: report of 110 cases, *Am J Surg* (1947) **74**:117–28.

3 Adler DD, Rebner M, Pennes DR, Accessory breast tissue in the axilla: mammographic appearance, *Radiology* (1987) **163**:709–11.

4 American Cancer Society, *News conference on mammography guidelines*, June 27, 1989.

5 Andersen JA, Carter D, Linell F, A symposium on sclerosing duct lesions of the breast, *Pathol Annu* (1986) **21**(2):145–79.

6 Andersen JA, Gram JB, Radial scar in the female breast. A long-term follow-up study of 32 cases, *Cancer* (1984) **53**:2557–60.

7 Andersson I, Mammography in clinical practice, *Medical Radiography and Photography* (1986) **62**:1–40.

8 Andersson I, Hildell J, Muhlow A et al, Number of projections in mammography: influence on detection of breast disease, *AJR* (1978) **130**:349–51.

9 Andersson I, Marsal L, Nilsson B et al, Abnormal axillary lymph nodes in rheumatoid arthritis, *Acta Radiol [Diagn]* (1980) **21**:645–9.

10 Arey LB, *Developmental anatomy: a textbook and laboratory manual of embryology*, 7th edn (Saunders: Philadelphia, 1965) 449–53.

11 Baker LH, Breast Cancer Detection Demonstration Project: five-year summary report, *CA* (1982) **32**:194–225.

12 Bassett LW, Bunnell DH, Jahanshahi R et al, Breast cancer detection: one versus two views, *Radiology* (1987) **165**:95–7.

13 Bassett LW, Gold RH, Breast radiography using the oblique projection, *Radiology* (1983) **149**:585–7.

14 Bassett LW, Gold RH, Cove HC, Mammographic spectrum of traumatic fat necrosis: the fallibility of 'pathognomonic' signs of carcinoma, *AJR* (1978) **130**:119–22.

15 Bassett LW, Gold RH, Mirra JM, Nonneoplastic breast calcifications in lipid cysts: development after excision and primary irradiation, *AJR* (1982) **138**:335–8.

16 Bassett LW, Kimme-Smith C, Sutherland LK et al, Automated and hand-held breast US: effect on patient management, *Radiology* (1987) **165**:103–8.

17 Berkowitz JE, Gatewood OMB, Donovan GV et al, Dermal breast calcifications: localization with template-guided placement of skin marker, *Radiology* (1987) **163**:282.

18 Berkowitz JE, Gatewood OMB, Gayler BW, Equivocal mammographic findings: evaluation with spot compression, *Radiology* (1989) **171**:369–71.

19 Bloomer WD, Berenberg AL, Weissman BN, Mammography of the definitively irradiated breast, *Radiology* (1976) **118**:425–88.

20 Bohman LG, Bassett LW, Gold RH et al, Breast metastases from extramammary malignancies, *Radiology* (1982) **144**:309–12.

21 Brenner RJ, Sickles EA, Acceptability of periodic follow-up as an alternative to biopsy for mammographically detected lesions interpreted as probably benign, *Radiology* (1989) **171**:645–6.

22 Bruwer A, Nelson GW, Spark RP, Punctate intranodal gold deposits simulating microcalcifications on mammograms, *Radiology* (1987) **163**:87–8.

23 Callen JP, Dermatomyositis, *Int J Dermatol* (1979) **18**:423–33.

24   Chaudary MA, Millis RR, Hoskins EO et al, Bilateral primary breast cancer: a prospective study of disease incidence, *Br J Surg* (1984) **71**:711–14.

25   Clayton F, Pure mucinous carcinomas of breast: morphologic features and prognostic correlates, *Hum Pathol* (1986) **17**:34–8.

26   Cole-Beuglet C, Goldberg BB, Kurtz AB et al, Ultrasound mammography: A comparison with radiographic mammography, *Radiology* (1981) **139**:693–8.

27   Collette HJ, Day NE, de Waard F et al, Evaluation of screening for breast cancer in a nonrandomized study (the DOM project) by means of a case-control study, *Lancet* (1984) **1**:1224–6.

28   Crothers JG, Butler NF, Fortt RW et al, Fibroadenolipoma of the breast, *Br J Radiol* (1985) **58**:191–202.

29   Czernobilsky B, Intracystic carcinoma of the female breast, *Surg Gynecol Obstet* (1967) **124**:93–8.

30   De Chonoky T, Augmentation mammoplasty: survey of complications in 10941 patients by 265 surgeons, *Plast Reconstr Surg* (1970) **45**:573–7.

31   de Paredes ES, *Atlas of film-screen mammography* (Urban & Schwarzenberg: Baltimore) 1989.

32   Dershaw DD, Chaglassian TA, Mammography after prosthesis placement for augmentation or reconstruction mammoplasty, *Radiology* (1989) **170**:69–74.

33   Dixon JM, Anderson TJ, Lumsden AB et al, Mammary duct ectasia, *Br J Surg* (1983) **70**:601–3.

34   Dixon JM, Anderson TJ, Page DL et al, Infiltrating lobular carcinoma of the breast, *Histopathology* (1982) **6**:149–61.

35   Dixon JM, Anderson TJ, Page DL et al, Infiltrating lobular carcinoma of the breast: an evaluation of the incidence and consequence of bilateral disease, *Br J Surg* (1983) **70**:513–16.

36   Dupont WD, Page DL, Risk factors for breast cancer in women with proliferative breast disease, *N Engl J Med* (1985) **312**:146–51.

37   Egan JF, Saylor CB, Goodman MJ, A technique for localizing occult breast lesions, *CA* (1976) **26**:32–7.

38   Egan RL, McSweeney MB, Intramammary lymph nodes, *Cancer* (1983) **51**:1838–42.

39   Egan RL, McSweeney MB, Sewell CW, Intramammary calcifications without an associated mass in benign and malignant diseases, *Radiology* (1980) **137**:1–7.

40   Eklund GW, Busby RC, Miller SH et al, Improved imaging of the augmented breast, *AJR* (1988) **151**:469–73.

41   Feig SA, Mammography equipment: principles, features, selection, *Radiol Clin North Am* (1987) **25**:897–911.

42   Feig SA, Shaber GS, Patchefsky A et al, Analysis of clinically occult and mammographically occult breast tumors, *AJR* (1977) **128**:403–8.

43   Feig SA, Shaber GS, Patchefsky A et al, Tubular carcinoma of the breast. Mammographic appearance and pathological correlation, *Radiology* (1978) **129**:311–14.

44   Fenoglio C, Lattes R, Sclerosing papillary proliferations in the female breast. A benign lesion often mistaken for carcinoma, *Cancer* (1974) **33**:691–700.

45   Fisher ER, Gregorio RN, Fisher B et al, The pathology of invasive breast cancer. A syllabus derived from findings of the National Surgical Adjuvant Breast Project (protocol no. 4), *Cancer* (1975) **36**:1–85.

46   Fisher ER, Palekar AS, Redman C et al, Pathologic findings from the National Surgical Adjuvant Breast Project (protocol no. 4). VI. Invasive papillary cancer, *Am J Clin Pathol* (1980) **73**:313–22.

47   Fisher ER, Sass R, Fisher B et al, Pathologic findings from the Surgical Adjuvant Breast Project (protocol no. 6) 1. Intraductal carcinoma (DCIS), *Cancer* (1986) **57**:197–208.

48   Fu YS, Maksem JA, Huban CA et al, The relationship of breast cancer morphology and estrogen receptor protein status. In: Fenoglio CM, Wolff M, eds. *Progress in surgical pathology*, Vol III (Masson: New York 1981) 65–76.

49   Gallager HS, Leis HP Jr, Snyderman RK et al, eds. *The breast* (Mosby: St Louis 1978).

50   Gefter WB, Friedman AK, Goodman RL, The role of mammography in evaluating patients with early carcinoma of the breast for tylectomy and radiation therapy, *Radiology* (1982) **142**:77–80.

51 Gershon-Cohen J, Moore L, Roentgeno-graphy of giant fibroadenoma of the breast (cystosarcoma phyllodes), *Radiology* (1960) **74**:619–25.

52 Gold RH, Montgomery CK, Rambo ON, Significance of margination of benign and malignant infiltrative mammary lesions: roentgenologic–pathologic correlation, *AJR* (1973) **118**:881–94.

53 Grow JL, Lewison EF, Superficial throm-bophlebitis of the breast, *Surg Gynecol Obstet* (1963) **126**:180–2.

54 Haagensen CD, *Diseases of the breast*, 3rd edn (Saunders: Philadelphia 1986).

55 Hajdu SI, Urban JA, Cancers metastatic to the breast, *Cancer* (1972) **29**:1691–6.

56 Hall FM, Storella JM, Silverstone DZ et al, Nonpalpable breast lesions: recommenda-tions for biopsy based on suspicion of carci-noma at mammography, *Radiology* (1988) **167**:353–8.

57 Harris JR, Recht A, Amalric R et al, Time course and prognosis of local recurrence following primary radiation therapy for early breast cancer, *J Clin Oncol* (1984) **53**:37–41.

58 Haskell CM, Cochran AJ, Barsky SH et al, Metastasis of unknown origin, *Curr Probl Cancer* (1988) **12**:5–58.

59 Hermann G, Schwartz IS, Focal fibrous dis-ease of the breast: mammographic detection of an unappreciated condition, *AJR* (1983) **140**:1245–6.

60 Hessler C, Schnyder P, Ozzello L, Hamar-toma of the breast: diagnostic observation of 16 cases, *Radiology* (1978) **126**:95–8.

61 Hilton SV, Leopold GR, Olson LK et al, Real-time breast sonography: application in 300 consecutive patients, *AJR* (1986) **147**:479–86.

62 Hoeffken W, Lanyi M, *Mammography: tech-nique, diagnosis, differential diagnosis, results* (Saunders: Philadelphia 1977).

63 Holland R, The role of specimen X-ray in the diagnosis of breast cancer, *Diagn Imaging Clin Med* (1985) **54**:178–85.

64 Homer MJ, Nonpalpable mammographic abnormalities: timing the follow-up studies, *AJR* (1981) **136**:923–6.

65 Homer MJ, Nonpalpable breast lesion loca-

lization using curved-end retractable wire, *Radiology* (1985) **157**:259–60.

66 Homer MJ, Cooper AG, Pile-Spellman ER, Milk of calcium in breast microcysts: man-ifestation as a solitary focal disease, *AJR* (1988) **150**:789–90.

67 Homer MJ, Pile-Spellman ER, Needle locali-zation of occult breast lesions with curved-end retractable wire: technique and pitfalls, *Radiology* (1986) **161**:547–8.

68 Consensus of Cancer Committee of the College of American Pathologists, Is 'fibro-cystic disease' of the breast precancerous? *Arch Pathol Lab Med* (1986) **110**:171–3.

69 Kalisher L, Xeroradiography of axillary lymph node disease, *Radiology* (1975) **115**:67–71.

70 Kalisher L, Chu AM, Peyster RG, Clinico-pathological correlations of xeroradiography in determining involvement of metastatic axillary nodes in female breast cancer, *Radiology* (1976) **121**:333–5.

71 Klein DL, Sickles EA, Effects of needle aspiration on the mammographic appear-ance of the breast: guide to the proper timing of the mammography examination, *Radiology* (1982) **145**:44.

72 Kline TS, Kannan V, Papillary carcinoma of the breast. A cytomorphic analysis, *Arch Pathol Lab Med* (1986) **110**:189–91.

73 Kobayashi T, Takatani O, Hattori N et al, Differential diagnosis of breast tumors. The sensitivity graded method of ultrasono-tomography and clinical evaluation of its diagnostic accuracy, *Cancer* (1974) **33**:940–51.

74 Kopans DB, DeLuca S, A modified needle-hookwire technique to simplify preoperative localization of occult breast lesions, *Radio-logy* (1980) **134**:781.

75 Kopans DB, Lindfors K, McCarthy KA et al, Spring hookwire breast lesion localizer: use with rigid-compression mammographic sys-tems, *Radiology* (1985) **157**:537–8.

76 Kopans DB, Meyer JE, Versatile spring hookwire breast lesion localizer, *AJR* (1982) **138**:586–7.

77 Kopans DB, Meyer JE, Homer MJ et al, Dermal deposits mistaken for breast calcifi-cations, *Radiology* (1983) **149**:592–4.

78 Kopans DB, Meyer JE, Lindfors KK, Whole-breast US imaging: four-year follow-up, *Radiology* (1985) **157**:505–7.

79 Kopans DB, Swann CA, White G et al, Asymmetric breast tissue, *Radiology* (1989) **171**:639–43.

80 Kraus FT, Neubecker RD, The differential diagnosis of papillary tumors of the breast, *Cancer* (1962) **15**:444–55.

81 Lane N, Göksel H, Salerno RA et al, Clinico-pathologic analysis of the surgical curability of breast cancers: a minimum two year study of a personal series, *Ann Surg* (1961) **153**:483–98.

82 Lanyi M, *Diagnosis and differential diagnosis of breast calcifications* (Springer-Verlag: New York 1988).

83 Leborgne R, Diagnosis of tumors of the breast by simple roentgenography: calcifications in carcinoma, *AJR* (1951) **65**:1–11.

84 Lesser ML, Rosen PP, Kinne DW, Multicentricity and bilaterality in invasive breast carcinoma, *Surgery* (1982) **91**:234–40.

85 Levitan LH, Witten DM, Harrison EG, Calcification in breast disease mammographic–pathologic correlation, *AJR Radium Therapy Nuc Med* (1964) **92**:29–39.

86 Libshitz HI, Montague ED, Paulus DD, Calcifications and the therapeutically irradiated breast, *AJR* (1977) **128**:1021–5.

87 Linden SS, Sickles EA, Sedimented calcium in benign breast cysts: the full spectrum of mammographic presentations, *AJR* (1989) **152**:967–71.

88 Lindfors KK, Kopans DB, McCarthy KA et al, Breast cancer metastases to intramammary lymph nodes, *AJR* (1986) **146**:133–6.

89 Linell F, Ljungberg O, Andersson I, Breast carcinoma. Aspects of early stages, progression and related problems, *Acta Pathol Microbiol Scand* (1980) **272A**(Supp):1–233.

90 Ljungqvist U, Andersson I, Hildell J et al, Mammary hamartoma, a benign breast lesion, *Acta Chir Scand* (1979) **145**:227–30.

91 Love SM, Gelman RS, Silen W, Sounding Board. Fibrocystic 'disease' of the breast—a nondisease? *N Engl J Med* (1982) **307**:1010.

92 Lundgren B, The oblique view at mammography, *Br J Radiol* (1977) **50**:626–8.

93 Lundgren B, Jakobsson S, Single view mammography. A simple and efficient approach to breast cancer screening, *Cancer* (1976) **38**:1124–9.

94 Mammography 1982: a statement of the American Cancer Society, *CA* (1982) **32**(4):226–31.

95 Mann BD, Giuliano AE, Bassett LW et al, Delayed diagnosis of breast cancer as a result of normal mammograms, *Arch Surg* (1983) **118**:23–4.

96 Martin JE, Moskowitz M, Milbrath J, Breast cancer missed by mammography, *AJR* (1979) **132**:737–9.

97 McDivitt RW, Breast cancer multicentricity. In: McDivitt RW, Obermann HA, Ozzello L, Kaufman N, eds. *The breast* (Williams & Wilkins: Baltimore 1984) 139–48.

98 McDivitt RW, Farrow JH, Stewart FW, Breast carcinoma arising in solitary fibro-adenomas, *Surg Gynecol Obstet* (1967) **125**:572–6.

99 McLelland R, Mammography 1984: challenge to radiology, *AJR* (1984) **143**:1–4.

100 Mendelson EB, Harris KM, Doshi N et al, Infiltrating lobular carcinoma: mammographic patterns with pathologic correlation, *AJR* (1989) **153**:265–71.

101 Millis RR, Davis R, Stacey AJ, The detection and significance of calcifications in the breast: a radiological and pathological study, *Br J Radiol* (1976) **49**:12–26.

102 Minagi H, Youker JE, Roentgen appearance of fat necrosis in the breast, *Radiology* (1968) **90**:62–5.

103 Moore OS Jr, Foote FW Jr, The relatively favorable prognosis of medullary carcinoma of the breast, *Br J Cancer* (1949) **2**:635–42.

104 Moskowitz M, Screening is not diagnosis, *Radiology* (1979) **133**:265–8.

105 Moskowitz M, The predictive value of certain mammographic signs in screening for breast cancer, *Cancer* (1983) **51**:1007–11.

106 Moskowitz M, Libshitz HI, Mammographic screening for breast cancer by lateral view only. Is it practical? *J Can Assoc Radiol* (1977) **28**:259–61.

107 Norris HJ, Taylor HB, Relationship of histologic features to behavior of cystosarcoma

phyllodes. Analysis of ninety-four cases, *Cancer* (1967) **20**:2090–9.

108 Page DL, Cancer risk assessment in benign breast biopsies, *Hum Pathol* (1986) **17**:871–4.

109 Page DL, Anderson TJ, *Diagnostic histopathology of the breast* (Churchill Livingstone: New York 1987).

110 Page DL, Dupont WD, Rogers LW et al, Intraductal carcinoma of the breast: follow-up after biopsy only, *Cancer* (1982) **49**:751–8.

111 Paulus DD, Malignant masses in the therapeutically irradiated breast, *AJR* (1980) **135**:789–95.

112 Paulus DD, Conservative treatment of breast cancer: mammography in patient selection and follow-up, *AJR* (1984) **143**:483–7.

113 Penn I, Brunson ME, Cancers after cyclosporine therapy, *Transplantation Proceedings* (1988) **20**:885–92.

114 Powell RW, McSweeney MB, Wilson CE, X-ray calcifications as the only basis for breast biopsy, *Ann Surg* (1983) **197**:555–9.

115 Rickert RR, Kalisher L, Hutter RVP, Indurative mastopathy: a benign sclerosing lesion of breast with elastosis which may simulate carcinoma, *Cancer* (1981) **47**:561–71.

116 Ridolfi RL, Rosen PP, Port A et al, Medullary carcinoma of the breast: a clinicopathologic study with 10-year follow-up, *Cancer* (1977) **40**:1365–85.

117 Rivera-Pomar JM, Villanova JR, Burgos-Bretones JJ et al, Focal fibrous disease of the breast, *Virchows Arch [Pathol Anat]* (1980) **386**:59–64.

118 Robbins GF, Berg JW, Bilateral primary breast cancer: a prospective clinicopathological study, *Cancer* (1964) **17**:1501–27.

119 Rosen PP, Kosloff C, Lieberman PH et al, Lobular carcinoma in situ of the breast. Detailed analysis of 99 patients with average follow-up of 24 years, *Am J Surg Pathol* (1978) **2**:225–51.

120 Rosner D, Bedwani RN, Vana J et al, Noninvasive breast carcinoma: results of a national survey by the American College of Surgeons, *Ann Surg* (1980) **192**:139–47.

121 Sadowsky N, Kopans DB, Breast cancer, *Radiol Clin North Am* (1983) **21**:51–65.

122 Sandison AT, Metastatic tumors in the breast, *Br J Surg* (1959) **47**:54–8.

123 Schneider JA, Invasive papillary breast carcinoma: mammographic and sonographic appearance, *Radiology* (1989) **171**:377–9.

124 Schwartz GF, Clinical implications of breast cancer risk factors. In: Feig SA, McClelland R, eds. *Breast carcinoma: current diagnosis and treatment* (Masson: New York 1983) 89–94.

125 Schwartz GF, Patchefsky AS, Feig SA et al, Clinically occult breast cancer, *Ann Surg* (1980) **191**:8–12.

126 Shapiro S, Venet W, Strax P et al, Ten to fourteen year effect of screening on breast cancer mortality, *J Natl Cancer Inst* (1982) **69**:349–55.

127 Sickles EA, Mammographic features of 'early' breast cancer, *AJR* (1984) **143**:461–4.

128 Sickles EA, Mammographic features of 300 consecutive nonpalpable breast cancers, *AJR* (1986) **146**:661–3.

129 Sickles EA, Breast calcifications: mammographic evaluation, *Radiology* (1986) **160**:289–93.

130 Sickles EA, Abele JS, Milk of calcium within tiny benign breast cysts, *Radiology* (1981) **141**:655–8.

131 Sickles EA, Filly RA, Callen PW, Breast cancer detection with ultrasonography and mammography: comparison using state-of-the-art equipment, *AJR* (1983) **140**:843–5.

132 Sickles EA, Filly RA, Callen PW, Benign breast lesions: ultrasound detection and diagnosis, *Radiology* (1984) **151**:467–70.

133 Sickles EA, Galvin HB, Breast arterial calcification with association with diabetes mellitus: too weak a correlation to have clinical utility, *Radiology* (1985) **155**:577–9.

134 Sickles EA, Herzog KA, Mammography of the postsurgical breast, *AJR* (1981) **136**:585–8.

135 Sickles EA, Klein DL, Goodson WH III et al, Mammography after needle aspiration of palpable breast masses, *Am J Surg* (1983) **145**:395–7.

136 Sickles EA, Weber WN, Galvin HB et al,

Baseline screening mammography: one vs two views per breast, *AJR* (1986) **147**:1149–53.

137   Silverberg E, Boring CC, Squires TS, Cancer statistics, 1990, *CA* (1990) **40**:9–26.

138   Snyder RE, Mammography and lobular carcinoma in situ, *Surg Obstet Gynecol* (1966) **22**:225–60.

139   Snyder RE, Specimen radiography and preoperative localization of nonpalpable breast cancer, *Cancer* (1980) **46**:950–6.

140   Stomper PC, Kopans DB, Sadowsky NL et al, Is mammography painful, a multicenter patient survey, *Arch Intern Med* (1988) **148**:5221–4.

141   Stomper PC, Recht A, Berenberg AL et al, Mammographic detection of recurrent cancer in the irradiated breast, *AJR* (1987) **148**:39–43.

142   Swann CA, Kopans DB, Koerner FC et al, Halo sign and malignant breast lesions, *AJR* (1987) **149**:1145.

143   Tabár L, Dean PB, *Teaching atlas of mammography*, 2nd edn (Thieme–Stratton: New York 1985).

144   Tabár L, Fagerberg CJ, Gad A et al, Reduction in mortality from breast cancer after mass screening with mammography. Randomized trial from the Breast Cancer Screening Working Group of the Swedish National Board of Health and Welfare, *Lancet* (1985) **1(8433)**:829–32.

145   Tabár L, Pántek Z, Dean PB, The diagnostic and therapeutic value of breast cyst puncture and pneumocystography, *Radiology* (1981) **141**:659–63.

146   Threatt B, Appleman H, Dow R et al, Percutaneous needle localization of clustered mammary microcalcifications prior to biopsy, *AJR* (1974) **121**:839–42.

147   Toombs BD, Kalisher L, Metastatic disease to the breast: clinical pathologic, and radiographic features, *AJR* (1977) **129**:673–6.

148   Troupin RH, Lobular carcinoma in situ—an incidental finding. Breast Imaging. In: Feig SA, ed. Categorical Course Syllabus of the 88th Annual Meeting of the ARRS (American Roentgen Ray Society, 1988) 79–88.

149   Urban JA, Bilaterality of cancer of the breast. Biopsy of the opposite breast, *Cancer* (1967) **20**:1867–70.

150   Verbeek AL, Hendricks HJ, Holland R et al, Reduction of breast cancer mortality through mass screening with modern mammography. First results of the Nijmegen project, 1975–1981, *Lancet* (1984) **1(8388)**:1222–4.

151   Wellings SR, A hypothesis of the origin of human breast cancer from the terminal ductal lobular unit, *Pathol Res Pract* (1980) **166**:515–35.

152   Wild JJ, Reid JM, Further pilot echographic studies on the histologic structure of tumors of the living intact human breast, *Am J Pathol* (1952) **28**:839–61.

153   Wolfe JN, *Xeroradiography: breast masses* (Thomas: Springfield 1977).

Index